HOW NOT TO BE SICK.

A SEQUEL TO "PHILOSOPHY OF EATING."

BY

ALBERT J. BELLOWS, M.D.,

AUTHOR OF "PHILOSOPHY OF EATING," LATE PROFESSOR OF CHEMISTRY, PHYSIOLOGY, HYGIENE, ETC.

TO "EAT TO LIVE" IS TO "LIVE TO EAT."

NEW YORK:
PUBLISHED BY HURD AND HOUGHTON.
Cambridge: Riverside Press.
1869.

PREFACE.

In "The Philosophy of Eating," to which this little volume is intended as a sequel, I have endeavored to establish the following propositions: —

That when, "In the beginning, God created the heaven and the earth," a plan was instituted and laws made by which in the soil of all the earth should be deposited all the elements of the human system, excepting those deposited in the atmosphere, and in the water, and by which the "grass, the herb yielding seed, and the fruit-tree yielding fruit after its kind," should take up these elements, and keep them in deposit, to be eaten directly by man, and thus furnish all the requisite elements to keep the system in repair; or to be eaten by animals, and be deposited in their flesh for the same purpose.

That no elements except those thus prepared are ever allowed to enter the composition of the human system, and that even these elements cease to be capable of assimilation as soon as the herb or the flesh that contains them becomes disorganized by decomposition; becoming, in that case, immediately poisonous. That these organized elements are mixed in the right proportions, varying only in their muscle-making, heat-producing, and brain-feeding elements, to adapt them to various conditions in regard to climate, physical, and mental exercise, &c., so that anywhere from the equator to the poles we find food adapted to our circumstances.

That in separating the muscle-making elements from the heating, as is done in the making of butter, fine flour, and sugar, we supply the system with too large a proportion of heating elements, and not only waste a large part of those expensive articles of food, but by keeping the temperature too high, predispose to and induce most of the inflammatory diseases to which we are subject.

That our unperverted tastes and appetites act in harmony with these laws, protecting the system from harm, promoting our enjoyment in keeping the commandments, and obeying our modified instincts.

That the different organs and functions require different elements of food, and have the power of taking from it, while circulating in the blood, these different elements, according to their requirements; and that no organ can perform its duties unless proper elements are thus supplied.

That some articles of food contain more and some less of the elements required under different circumstances; so that, by a table of analyses of the different articles, comparing them with the demands of the different organs and functions, under different circumstances, we can at any time adjust our diet to our circumstances.

If these propositions are established, — and in over two hundred reviews or notices of the book by editors or literary men, not solicited or paid for, not one of them has been controverted or denied, — there must be many important practical inferences to be drawn from them pertaining to the choice of food for different classes of people, under their varied circumstances, and pertaining to the prevention and cure of the various diseases to which we are subject in consequence of bad food, bad cooking, &c.

Some of these inferences are drawn in the text-book, and will be found under the heads — Bread-making; Professor Horsford's Phosphatic Bread; French Plan of Bread-making; Analysis of the different Kinds of Food in common Use; the loss of strengthening Elements in fine Flour, Butter, and Sugar; Food for the Brain and Nerves; Food for Precocious Children; Food for Old People; Food for Children; How to purify the Blood; Value of Pure Water; Uses and Abuses of Alcoholic Drinks, Wines, Tea, and Coffee; The Value of the Principle which gives Relish to Food, &c.; Bathing and Friction of the Skin; Use of Condiments, &c.

But having received numerous requests that its principle might be carried out more in detail on practical subjects, the "HOW NOT TO BE SICK" is the answer.

NO. 90 SPRINGFIELD STREET,
BOSTON, Nov., 1868.

A. J. B.

CONTENTS.

PAGE

Thinking Men, Food for. 11
Laboring Men, Food for. 22
Economy in using Natural Food. 42
Gustatory Enjoyment, how obtained. 44
Sedentary People, Food for. 51
Winter, Food for. 56
Chronic Diseases cured by Diet. 60
Summer, Food for. 66
Dyspepsia, prevented and cured by Diet. 69
Smell, a Guardian Angel. 82
Taste, a Guardian Angel. 86
Consumption, prevented and cured by Diet. 91
Inflammations, prevented and cured by Diet. 128
Animal Food, is it injurious?. 136
Medical Hobbies. 138
Consumption of the Blood. 142
Vigilance the price of Health. 151
Apoplexy and Neuralgia prevented and cured by Diet. . 157
Teeth defective, how prevented by Diet. 161
Heart Diseases, prevented and cured by Diet. . . . 176
Corpulence, prevented and cured by Diet. 181
Leanness, prevented and cured by Diet. 190
Medicines, their Uses and Abuses. 203
Doctors, why they differ. 209
"Currents and Counter Currents in Medical Science." . . 232
Crusade against Homeopathy. 247
City Hospital. 256
Medicines a Gift from God. 279
Three Systems of Practice of Medicine. 285
Domestic Practice. How to select Medicines. 308
Virtues of twenty principal Medicines for Families. . . 326
Sun-stroke, its Cause and Prevention. 333
Poisons from Water Pipes, Cooking Utensils, Bread, &c. . 345
Galvanic Action dissolving Metals in every Kitchen. . . 356
Gout, prevented and cured by Diet. 344
Grecian Bend. 361

PAGE
Acids needed every Day. 20
Aconite. Arsenicum. 326
Agassiz on Fish Diet. 13
Animal Food, is it injurious? 136
Apoplexy, its Cause and Prevention. 157
Appetite, how always to be good. 193–195
Atmosphere, how made impure. 93

Banting, the fat Englishman. 61, 186
Beans and Peas, Nutriment in them. 29
Blood impure, the Cause of Consumption. . . 93, 142
Blood, how to purify it. 147–149
Breath, why not always sweet. 197
Bladder, Inflammation of. 315
Belladonna, Bryonia, Baptisia. 327

Curse for Adam's Transgression. 14
Chamomilla, Colocynth, Collinsonia. 328
Cheese, strengthening Power of. 19, 26
Corn, Southern, more strengthening than Northern. . . 28
Climate, Adaptation of Food to. 57
Cheese, Effects of, in excessive Quantities. 62
Children, their Tastes perverted the first Day of Life. . . 72
Consumption, its Causes. 91, 94, 95, 96
from compressing the Chest. 95, 104
from eating heating Food. 96, 106
from low-neck Dresses. 97, 105
from crude Medicines. 98
from bad Air. 93
why most prevalent in cold Climates. 94
made worse by Whiskey, Cod-liver Oil, heating Food, &c. 99
made worse by Iron, Phosphorus, and all crude Drugs. . 98
hereditary not necessarily fatal. 113
may be prevented, and may be cured. . . . 114, 124
danger of a vacillating Course of Treatment. . . 117
danger of erroneous Teachings. 120
Constipations, Cathartics. 318
Croup, how to treat it. 314
Corpulence, may be cured philosophically. 181
Banting's Method of Cure defective. 186
Examples of Cure. 185
the Principle of Cure. 182
Cheerfulness promotes Digestion. 201

PAGE
Crusade against Homeopathy. 247
Crusade Number Two. 253
Cramps and Colics, how cured. 316

Diseases cured by Diet. 60
Diseases of the Heart produced by Cheese. 62
Dyspepsia, its Cause and Cure. 69
  Animals in their natural State exempt from it. . . 71
  Infants have it on the first Day of Life. . . . 72
  how it is developed by wrong Diet. 73
  how it may be cured. 75
Digestion, the Process of. 73, 199
Doctors differ, how then decide? 225
Drugs always do Harm. 204, 227, 280
Dose of Medicine. 224
Dangerous Neighbors. 283
Domestic Practice, Books, &c. 310
Diphtheria, Treatment of. 314
Diarrhœa and Dysentery, how to be treated. . . . 317

Economy of eating natural Food. 42
Errors, dangerous. 123
Eating slowly important. 200
  too much, how avoided. 33
  how to enjoy it. 44, 75
Experiments on the Sick dangerous and useless. . 210–212

Fruits, Nourishment in them. 20
  how to be kept the Year round. 79
  important in warm Weather. 67
  their Acids are necessary every Day. 20
Farmers, how degenerated. 25
Fish, furnishes Food for the Brain. 13
  why Trouts are better than Eels. 16
  are phosphatic Food. 12
  wants carbonaceous Elements. 31
Food, Variety necessary. 36
  what Combination necessary daily. 38
  containing Excess of muscle-making Elements. . . 39
  containing Excess of carbonaceous Elements. . . 40
  how to relish it. 197
  how wasted. 24
  the Pleasures of eating natural Food. 44
  why to be eaten slowly. 199

PAGE
Food, why to be eaten cheerfully. 202
why to be eaten at regular Times. 193
Flavor, how preserved in cooking. 53
Fixed Principles important in Sickness. 305
Flour the principal Source of excessive Heat. . . . 40
Fermentation, how to prevent it. 79

Gout, Prevention and Cure of. 339
Gladiators lived on Barley. 22
Greenland, Food in. 57
Gelseminum. 38
Grecian Bend. 361

Horses, how trained. 22
Habits, wrong, perpetuated. 49
Hernia cured by Diet. 61
Hobbies, medical. 152
Health, how to preserve it. 176
Hereditary Diseases, how transmitted. 174
Heart, Diseases of, how cured. 176
Homeopathy, is it reasonable? 221
effects of Medicines. 232
misrepresented. 236
Old School Doctors practise it. 239
no Deception in it. 243
how it was to be killed in an Hour. 247
and Allopathy, the Difference between them. . . . 267–270
in France. 272
opinions of learned Men respecting it. 268
its present Condition in Europe. 250
the Effect of Opposition to it in Boston. 277
Hahnemann's Ghost. 252
Hospital, Report of, by Dr. Lawrence. 259
Hospital, the Contest of Doctors. 271
Heroic Treatment. 285
High and Low Dilutions. 295–300
Headaches, how cured. 320
Hepar Sulphur, Hippocastanum, and Hydrastes, as Medicines. 329

Inflammations, how to be treated. 128, 313
Iron dangerous as Medicine. 143
Infinitesimal Atoms produce Disease. 298
Ipecac, its Uses as a Medicine. 329

PAGE
Laboring Men, Food for. 22
Lungs, Structure of. 92
Life, how to prolong it. 153
Leanness, how prevented and how cured. 190
Law of Cure. 214
Louse drowned in a Lake. 232

Meats, the Lean of. 29
give Strength according to the Activity of the Animal. . 16
Mould always dangerous. 84
Medicines, how to avoid them. 107
how to select them. 112, 308
their Uses and Abuses. 218
a Gift from God. 279
the Virtues of such as are needed in Families. . 328–331
domestic Use of. 309
Mothers sacrifice their Children. 50, 165, 283
nursing and expectant, responsible for the Defects of their Children. 162, 163
Mercurius, what it is used for. 329

Neuralgia, how to relieve it. 319–330
Nux Vomica, its Use as a Medicine. 329

Phosphates in Food promote vital Action. 16
in raising Bread poisonous. 347
are lost in cooking. 18
in Consumption dangerous. 120
Parents, Responsibility of. 46
Poison from Copper. 346
from Lead. 346
from Zinc. 346
from Iron. 346
from Phosphorus. 347
from Galvanic Action. 346
in Lead Pipes. 346
in Boilers and Cisterns. 346
in Cooking Utensils. 346
in Bread. 347
in other Food. 346
Pigs have clean Mouths. 196
Practice of Medicine, three Modes. 205, 206
Persecution, its practical Effects. 277

PAGE
Pleurisy, how to be treated. 314
Prize-fighters, how prepare themselves. 22
Phytolacca, Podophylon, Pulsatilla, as Medicines. . . . 330

Review of Dr. Lawrence's Report. 265
Rheumatism, how treated. 115

Quack, what is a. 254

Sermons made on fat Pork. 12
Soldiers' Rations. 32
Sedentary People, Food for. 51
Scrofulous Sores cured by Diet. 64
Summer, Food for. 66
Smell, a Guardian Angel. 84
Sugar, &c., how they injure the Teeth. 166
Systems of Practice compared. 216, 303
Statistics of Diseases treated differently. 218, 269
Sickness, what to do first in. 313
Sticta as a Medicine. 331
Sun-stroke, its Cause and Prevention. 333

Thinking Men, Food for. 11
Teeth, how to secure good Teeth for Children. . . 165
defective for want of Nourishment. 164
Mothers responsible for the Teeth of their Children. . 165
bad Teeth hereditary. 173
injured by carbonaceous Food. 26
Taste, a Guardian Angel. 86
Taste perverted. 102
Treatment, expectant, or Nature-trusting. 287
Tonsils swelled, how treated. 314
Tartarized Antimony as a Medicine. 331

Veratrum as a Medicine. 331
Vegetable Food, Effects of. 137
Vigilance the Price of Health. 151
Vacillation in Practice dangerous. 307

Wheat, four hundred Varieties of. 15
Winter, Food for. 56
Water, how to get it pure. 80

HOW NOT TO BE SICK.

A SEQUEL TO "PHILOSOPHY OF EATING."

FOOD FOR THINKING MEN.

THAT one set of principles in food enables us to use the muscles, that another set enables us to keep up the animal heat, and another promotes the action of the brain and nerves, and enables us to think, I have endeavored to show. (See Philosophy of Eating, pages 16 and 17.)

That phosphorus is used up in thinking, as nitrogen is used in working the muscles, and carbon in furnishing animal heat and fat, I think has also been clearly demonstrated. (Philosophy of Eating, page 87.)

This idea, though not new to physiologists, has never been made practical, and, indeed, I have seen no attempt to develop it either for philosophical or practical purposes.

Vauqualin and L'Harittee, two celebrated French chemists, laid the foundation of its development in their analyses of the human brain, proving, as they did, that the brains of infants and idiots contain less than half the phosphorus that is found in the brains of men of common intellect, and that the proportion of phosphorus found was in proportion to the intellect; but for more than a quarter of a century it has remained without development or practical application.

Meantime it has also been proved by analysis of the secretions, that the more active the brain, the more phosphorus is used up and thrown off by the system, clergymen using up more on Sunday, and lawyers on court days, than at other times. And yet our professional men have lived as other men live, — eating what has come before them, without considering whether the elements they take are adapted to develop stupidity or mental vigor; eating, perchance, such stupefying articles as ham, or fat pork, and white bread and butter, while making or preaching a sermon, and such phosphatic food as trouts and other fish, with unbolted bread, vegetables, and fruits, when idle and rusticating. But a little observation would show a vast difference in the quality of sermons whether made and preached on carbonaceous or phosphatic diet; and the estimate of the old divine, "of the number of tons of beans and pork preached to in New England every Sunday, while the owners were asleep," might be offset by an estimate of the number of congregations, not only in New England, but in Old England, and all the rest of the fat and starch eating world, who are put asleep by sermons made from stupefying principles extracted from fat pork, fat beef, and superfine flour. (Philosophy of Eating, pages 16 and 17.)

The principle that mental activity depends on phosphatic food, I have been gratified to notice, has been recently endorsed by Professor Agassiz, in his address before the committee of the legislature of Massachusetts on the propagation and preservation of fishes.

He said, as reported in the Boston Journal, "The fish enters largely into the requisition of the human system. It is a kind of food which refreshes the system, especially after intellectual fatigue. There is no other article of food that supplies the waste of the head so thoroughly as fish diet; and the evidence of it is in the fact that all the inhabitants of the sea shores, the world over, are the brighter population of the country. Fish contains phosphorus to a large extent, — a chemical element which the brain requires for growth and health. He would not say that an exclusive use of fish would make a blockhead a wise man; but that the brain should not be wanting in one of its essential elements."

But man cannot live on fish alone, that food being generally deficient in carbonaceous elements to furnish animal heat; and we need a variety of food, one article being adapted to supply the deficiencies of others; and everywhere in the habitable world nature has furnished this variety, adapting it to different climates, tastes, constitutions, employments, and habits of life. For every animal but man appropriate food is placed, already cooked and prepared for digestion, within the reach of every species, in its own limited sphere, and its instincts direct with unerring certainty to the food best adapted to its development and health; but man, having intellect, is expected to use it in studying the wants of the system, and in analyzing food to ascertain its adaptedness to supply those wants, in the destitute condition in which he is placed, as implied in the sentence, "Cursed is the ground for thy sake: in sorrow shalt thou eat of it all the days of thy life; thorns also and thistles shall it bring forth to thee; and thou shalt eat the herb of the field. In the sweat of thy face shalt thou eat bread till thou return unto the ground."

Differ as we may in regard to the meaning of this passage, we find man in a condition in regard to food very different from that of other animals. Instead of having everything ready at his hand, he must cultivate the herbs, and the grasses, and tuberous roots, the grains, and vegetables, and fruits, and every luxury must be obtained by dint of his wits and his industry. All he finds growing spontaneously are a few berries and small imperfect fruits, and perhaps the juices of some plants and vegetables; everything else must be cooked and prepared to be capable of digestion and of furnishing nourishment, — all our delicious apples, and peaches, and grapes, and other fruit, are brought to the perfection in which we now find them by cultivation from these berries and small imperfect natural fruits. And all our grains and succulent plants and vegetables, which are our main dependences for food, are cultivated from the seeds of grasses, and from plants so unlike these excellent articles, that the origin of many of them, though doubtless still growing wild, is not recognized. For interesting examples of this change, wrought in many common articles of food, see Philosophy of Eating, pages 299–305.

To assist in selecting articles of food with suitable proportions of elements for muscles and brains, under different conditions and occupations in life, you will find analyses of about fifty articles, embracing most if not all articles of food in common use in the civilized world, in Philosophy of Eating, pages 121–125.

They are selected with great care, from English, French, German, and American analyses, but cannot in the nature of the case be positively, but only proximately correct; for no two specimens of any article, growing on different soils and in different climates, are found to contain precisely the same elements in the same proportions. For example: Of the four hundred different varieties of wheat, described and analyzed by the French Academy of Arts and Sciences, no two are found to contain the same elements in precisely the same proportions. Still, as a means of comparing one kind of grain and food with others, and of adapting them to our particular conditions and circumstances in life, these tables cannot fail to be practically valuable to any one who shall give attention to them.

It will be seen that in ordinary circumstances of temperature, muscular and mental exercise, &c., the proportions required are about fifteen per cent. of the nitrates, or muscle-making elements, to sixty-five to seventy of carbonates, or heat-producing elements, and two or three per cent. of phosphates, or food for brains and nerves, or a little more than four times as much carbonaceous food as nitrogenous, while the proportion of phosphates vary much, and are to be used more or less according to mental and physical activity, and that the proportions of these different elements are various in different articles, giving a wide field for selection and adaptation. And in the selection of animal food, it is of great practical use also to recur to the principles explained. (Philosophy of Eating, pages 82–90.)

The amount of phosphatic food contained in the flesh of any animal, and the physical and mental activity imparted by it, is in exact proportion to the activity of that animal, the flesh of the trout, pickerel, or salmon imparting much more mental and physical vigor than that of the dormant pout, eel, or flounder, and the flesh of the wild bison or hog more than that of the domestic ox or hog of the same species, and of the active working ox more than that of the dormant hog or calf, which are fed and fattened in a pen, without exercise. And the same remark holds true in relation to the flesh of wild and domestic fowls.

Without going to tables of analysis, therefore, much assistance can be had in selecting food for the brain by reference to this principle.

In comparing these various articles of food, with a view to determine their adaptation to our particular circumstances, the considerations mentioned in Philosophy of Eating, page 123, and elsewhere, must be noticed.

Neither the comparative proportions of heat-giving, muscle-making, or brain-feeding elements are exactly indicated by the carbonates, nitrates, or phosphates of the tables; the heating and fattening power of butter, and the fat of animals, being two and one half times greater than those of starch and sugar, and fibrin and casein giving greater muscular power than albumen, while the different effects of the different phosphates are still more important, as is shown by the table of analysis. (Philosophy of Eating, page 123.)

Phosphates of potash and soda furnish the brain and nerve power, while phosphates of lime and magnesia furnish the basis of the bones, so that in this respect these tables of analysis only approximate to the practical truth. They are, however, sufficiently accurate for the common duties of life; but for thinking men the following considerations are necessary.

On page 16, Philosophy of Eating, it is intimated that the phosphates should be subdivided into soluble and insoluble phosphates, and this for thinking men is an important distinction, both as it relates to the selection of food and its preservation and preparation. Take for example, beef or fish, which contain both soluble phosphates for the brain and insoluble phosphates for the bones. In pickling in brine, or in boiling, the soluble phosphates and much of the albumen are lost in the water, and of course boiled or salted beef or fish is not suitable food for the thinking man, although, retaining as it does the insoluble phosphates and fibrin, it may be good food for the laboring man. And the same considerations enter into the question of cooking or preparing all meats and vegetables.

The nitrates and phosphates of all meats and vegetables are partly soluble and partly insoluble, and therefore in soaking in cold water, all lose much that is important, especially to the thinking man. In cold water, albumen is dissolved or lost, but in hot water the albumen is coagulated, and mostly retained; but in hot water as well as cold the soluble phosphates are lost. Neither fish, nor meats, nor vegetables should therefore ever be pickled in brine, nor should they be boiled, unless in a little water, as in the admirable arrangement of Zimmermann or Duncklee, where all the soluble materials, as well as all the flavor, are retained in the water that is necessary to keep up the steam, and being used as gravy or soup, all the elements are saved, as nature intended.

In roasting also, or broiling, or indeed in any manner of cooking, care must be taken not to burn up or otherwise destroy or lose any of the juices of either vegetable or animal food; especially is this important for thinking men and for those whose digestion is feeble, the power of the stomach as well as the power of the brain being dependent on soluble phosphorus. And especially is the power of the stomach dependent on the flavor of food, as elsewhere shown. Let any one try the experiment of cooking meats, fish, potatoes, carrots, turnips, or any other food, animal or vegetable, in a steamer in which the flavor and all the steam are distilled back and saved, and compare the taste of them with that of the same food cooked so that all these elements are lost, and he will be astonished at the difference in flavor, digestibility, and mental and physical energy imparted by it.

Other articles of food may be wholesome to the laboring man, that are not wholesome to the thinking man. Cheese, for example, is very strengthening to bones and muscles, containing not only the concentrated nitrates of the milk, but also a large share of its phosphates; but the phosphates are mostly insoluble, the soluble phosphates having gone off in the whey. Cheese, therefore, while it may be excellent food for the laboring man, and for children whose bones are feeble, is too indigestible, and contains too little food for the brain, to be very valuable to the sedentary thinking man, especially as it tends to constipation, containing as it does almost no waste material. But with this exception, all articles of common food, cooked so as to retain their natural elements, are useful to thinking men in proportion to the phosphates indicated in the tables, containing, as they all do in their natural condition, soluble as well as insoluble phosphorus.

Of the amount of soluble phosphorus in animal food, we can judge, as I have before mentioned, without an analysis, by the degree of activity of the animal, as only soluble phosphorus gives either activity of brain or muscle; but of the soluble phosphorus in vegetable food we have to judge by a different estimate. The phosphates of succulent vegetables and fruits, when nourishment is mostly in their juices, are of course mostly soluble, and as their solid material is mostly woody fibre, and indigestible, they also furnish waste, which is very important to sedentary men, inclined as they are to constipation. They also contain the acids which are needed every day, especially in sedentary men, the action of whose liver is sluggish, to eliminate effete matters, which, if retained in the system, produce inaction of the brain, and indeed of the whole system, causing jaundice, sleepiness, scurvy, and troublesome diseases of the skin. Acid fruits and succulent vegetables are needed therefore every day of the year, especially in summer, and in winter by those who live in warm rooms, without much exercise; and the amount of refreshing nourishment in them is much greater than would at first appear by the tables of analysis. As they contain from seventy-five to ninety-seven per cent. of water, and only from three to twenty-five per cent. of solid matter, the per cent. of nitrogenous and phosphatic nourishment is greater than in more solid food in proportion to the amount of water.

For example: In wheat there is eighty-six per cent. of solid matter, of which fifteen per cent. is nitrogenous and about two per cent. is phosphatic. In apples there is but sixteen per cent. of solid matter, of which five per cent. is nitrogenous and one per cent. is phosphatic, so that in apples there is nearly twice the food for muscles; and, considering that in wheat the phosphates are partly insoluble, there is more than four times the food for the brain in apples than in wheat. And this estimate is not unfair, because there is as much water used in the digestion of wheat as in that of apples, all that is needed in the wheat being demanded and taken as drink. In other fruits and vegetables the proportionate amount of nitrates and phosphates is still greater, and it can readily be understood why, in warm weather, when carbonaceous food is not much needed, fruits and vegetables are so plentifully provided, and why they furnish such healthful action of the system and such vigor of mind.

FOOD FOR LABORING MEN.

THAT muscular power and activity is greater under the use of some kinds of food than others has been known and recorded for more than two thousand years. Before the Christian era the gladiators were so constantly trained on barley bread that they were called *hordearii*, hordeum being the Greek name for barley. And if we look at the analysis of barley (Philosophy of Eating, page 121), we shall see that it contains more nitrogenous, as well as more phosphatic elements, than wheat, or any other grain adapted to bread-making. Prize-fighters and professional pedestrians prepare themselves and sustain their extraordinary powers of action and endurance on the muscles of the ox or sheep and on unbolted bread. Horses, also, are trained for the race on food containing a large proportion of nitrogenous and phosphatic elements, as oats, barley, the bran of wheat, or Southern corn — never on Northern corn or fine wheat flour, which tend to fatness, but not to strength and activity. Indeed, the experience of practical men the world over corroborates the important truths developed by analyses of different articles of food, and the scientific inferences deduced from them ; and the tables found in Philosophy of Eating, pages 121–125, are therefore confidently referred to, for the purpose of assisting laboring men to determine what kind of food will give most muscular strength, and what, in the common way of living, is lost.

It will be seen that most of the kinds of natural food, as the meats of our domestic animals, fat and lean together, with unbolted wheat, potatoes, vegetables, milk, corn, rye, barley, &c., contain a due proportion of food for the muscles, nerves, and for animal heat, without the addition of such heating materials as fine flour, bread, butter, fat pork, or lard. And as neither of these last-named articles contain any, or but little of any, strength or life-giving elements, it follows, that, used with the food containing the natural mixture and proportions of all the elements required, these heating elements, not being wanted, are either thrown off and wasted, or, by increasing the amount of heat and by embarrassing the system, tend to produce inflammations and disease. But it will also be seen that other valuable articles, as beans and peas, and many fruits and vegetables, not containing enough of these carbonaceous materials, do require with them, or at the same meal, some butter, or other fat, or starch, or sugar, to give them the requisite heating power, especially in cold weather. A little attention to these tables, and the principles upon which they are made, would be of great service, not only for the preservation of health and strength, but for economy.

It will be noticed that the kinds of food most wasted, because eaten when not wanted by the system, are the most expensive. The article most used when not wanted, in Boston, is superfine flour, out of which has been bolted a large portion of its nitrates and phosphates. (See Philosophy of Eating, pages 25 and 26.) This being used with butter and sugar, furnishes very little but heating materials. The next article on which most money is expended and wasted, because most used with other articles containing enough of carbonaceous elements, is butter, which contains not a particle of strength or life-giving material, and therefore is never useful, except with food deficient in carbon.

And another article most extensively used, and, for the same reason, wasted, is sugar, which, though useful with too acid fruits, and as a part of a meal in which is too large a proportion of nitrogenous food, is worse than useless in confectionery, cakes, &c., especially if eaten between meals, and when food is not wanted, as it not only adds to the superfluous heat, but causes fermentation in the stomach and bowels, and causes, or tends to cause, flatulence, colic, dyspepsia, and the thousand and one troubles of the digestive organs, which we are apt to impute to green vegetables and fruit, when the fact is, these extra carbonaceous substances, in their passage out of the system, embarrass the digestion of natural food, and cause it to give us these troubles; and this is proved by the fact that those who avoid these expensive and useless articles may eat as much as they choose of green vegetables and fruits, and it gives them no flatulence, and produces no irritation.

Our puritanic forefathers, who lived on beans, peas,

unbolted grains, and the meats, vegetables, and fruits as they came from their fields and gardens, cooked in the simple manner best calculated to develop their natural flavor and prepare them for digestion, were not troubled with flatulence, colic, indigestion, &c. And our foremothers were not the pale-faced, flabby-muscled, toothless, chlorotic, consumptive, and sentimental race, as are their degenerate daughters of the present generation. Having plenty of nitrogen for the muscles, lime and silex for the teeth, iron for the blood, and all strength-giving articles of food for the lungs and digestive organs, and phosphorus for the brain, in natural food as God had furnished it, and their systems not being heated up and embarrassed by the extra carbonaceous food furnished in superfine flour, butter, and sugar, on which our daughters try, but fail, to live, they had all the elements necessary to promote the vigorous health of every organ and faculty, and none of the extra carbon which heats up the system, embarrasses the digestive organs, and renders us more liable to disease and less able to resist it.

Even our farmers, and their wives and daughters, have become terribly degenerated. Instead of the robust and healthy men, and the full-chested, healthy, rosy-cheeked, beautiful women, of former generations, we see a people almost as feeble and sickly as city people. And the reason is apparent. The outer crust of the wheat, and the buttermilk, which contain the nitrogen, phosphorus, and iron on which strength and energy, mental and physical, and beauty of complexion, depend, is given to the cattle and pigs, while they take themselves, instead, the butter, fine flour and sugar, which contain only the heating and disease-producing carbonates.

The robust Irishmen and Scotchmen, also, who come here with strong, energetic muscles, and sound teeth, from their oatmeal, wheat, and barley cakes, with their potatoes, buttermilk, and cheese, soon fall into our starch and grease eating habits, and become, or at least their children become, as pale, puny, and toothless as pure-blooded Yankees. Indeed, bringing with them, as they do, especially the laboring Irish, their clannish and unclean habits, and therefore breathing air impregnated with impurities, they suffer much more and die much faster than Yankees, whose habits of life, in this respect, are better. (See statements and statistics, in another chapter, relating to length of life, &c.)

Articles of Food best adapted to impart Muscular Power.

Cheese.

By the tables of analysis, so often referred to, it will be seen that cheese contains more elements of strength to the muscles and bones than any other article in common use in this country or in England. It contains from sixty to seventy per cent. of nitrogenous matter, and seven per cent. of phosphatic, to only nineteen of carbonaceous; and the phosphates being of the insoluble or bone-making class, it imparts strength to the bones and working power, in a more concentrated form than any other known article of food; and, being hard of digestion, it has also the good quality of staying by, or holding on, or, as the farmers say of salt beef and beans, "it is a good prop to lean over when at work." But it is not natural food, being only a part of the natural food, milk. It therefore needs additional elements to make it wholesome for a single meal. By a calculation made elsewhere, it will be seen that to eat three times a day we should require, at one meal, less than two ounces of food for the muscles. And we find that two ounces would be contained in three ounces of cheese, whereas, to produce the natural distention, nearly eight times as much bulk of food is required; and, therefore, on a meal of cheese sufficient to supply muscular power, the stomach would collapse into a condition in which the gastric juice could not be properly produced, and the digestive process could not go on. Then, again, in three ounces of cheese only one ounce of carbonaceous food would be produced, whereas there should be at least twelve ounces, to give its natural proportions. Then, again, in cheese there is almost no waste, and therefore cheese alone would produce fatal constipation in a very short time. Cheese, therefore, to be wholesome, must be eaten in small quantities, and, to get appropriate carbonaceous food, must be eaten with bread; and for this purpose white bread would not be objectionable, if it contained the requisite waste. If, therefore, we ate three ounces of cheese and three fourths of a pound of wheat bread, we should get nearly half the nitrates and carbonates needed for twenty-four hours, and in about the right proportions. But still we should get no waste, and only a part of the phosphatic elements needed; but with the addition of apples, or other fruits, or coarse bread, to supply the deficient elements, cheese would be excellent and cheap food for the laboring man.

Southern Corn.

Next to cheese, the long, tooth-shaped Southern corn, such as is delineated in Philosophy of Eating, page 25, figure 3, contains most nitrogen and phosphorus, compared with its carbon; and its phosphates being partly soluble, and its nitrogen in the form of albumen and gluten instead of casein, it is more easily digested, and it imparts more vigor and activity than cheese, and is therefore better adapted to work requiring rapidity of motion, but less continuous action than that to which cheese is adapted. It requires some addition of carbon, having but one part of nitrogenous to three of carbonaceous elements, whereas there is need of one to four in warm weather, and one to five in cold. It is, therefore, appropriately eaten with molasses, or meats, fat and lean; and even the negro diet of "hog and hominy" is not a bad one, especially in cool weather.

Beans and Peas.

Next come beans and peas, which, being very nearly alike in their proportions of necessary elements, will be considered together. They also contain too large a proportion of muscle-making principles, having twenty-four per cent. of nitrates to seventy of carbonates, and three to four per cent. of phosphates, partly soluble and partly insoluble, so that if we retain the liquor in which they are cooked, as in bean porridge or pea soup, they are good articles not only for laboring men but for thinking men, if they have good digestive powers. These also require additional carbon, and are appropriately eaten with butter, or fat pork and potatoes, with more of the vegetable carbonates in summer and of the animal in winter.

Lean Flesh of Meats.

Lean meats, or muscles of animals, contain about the same proportion of nitrates and phosphates as beans and peas, but they contain no carbonates at all, or at least the gelatine in them, which is carbonaceous, is not digestible, but is used as waste, to keep the bowels in action, gelatine in meats answering the same purpose as woody fibre answers in vegetable food. It is gelatine which gives consistence to soups, especially those made of joints of meat, and many people are deceived by the idea that the more gelatinous the more nourishing the soup; but nourishment comes from other elements. Still, to old people, and sedentary people who are inclined to costiveness, they are wholesome and valuable, and the gelatine performs an important office in the promotion of health.

The lean of beef contains twenty-five per cent. of food for muscles, seventy-five per cent. being water and waste. It is, if tender, very easily digested while fresh, and hard-working men prefer that which has been salted, as it "stays by" better; and as all the insoluble phosphates and all the fibrine is retained, it is good food for them, although the soluble phosphates and the albumen are lost in the brine. Lean meat can never, of course, be eaten alone, not having in it the necessary carbon to keep up steam to run the machine, but requires either fat or starch to supply the lungs with fuel, more or less according to temperature, &c., fat being best adapted to supply its carbonates in winter and starch in summer; and if fruits are eaten with meat, sugar also may be eaten without injury. Sugar seems to accord with vegetable diet rather than animal. There seems, however, to be required, to keep the system in good order, some variety, containing some fat, some starch, and some sugar; but it is always better to get these principles combined with food in Nature's own way, rather than in the concentrated form in which we find them in lard, butter, fine flour, and sugar; and the more nearly we conform to Nature's arrangements in this respect, as in all others, the better every way.

Fish.

The only other article of food in common use, in which the nitrates and phosphates are in excess of the carbonates, are the common varieties of fish in our climate. The only available carbon in fish is in the fat, of which, in most species, indeed in all species used as food in this country or England, there is but little, the gelatine, of which in many species there is a large proportion, being used for the same purpose as gelatine in red meat. It is carbonaceous, but not digestible, but serves the valuable purpose of keeping the bowels in order. The carbonates necessary to keep up the steam must, in a fish diet, be furnished either in butter, the fat of other animals, or in the starch of vegetables and grains, of which, perhaps, the potato furnishes the most valuable supply. Fish is more easily digested than red meat, but it gives less muscular power. It is not, therefore, satisfactory to those whose labor consists in lifting or steady muscular exertion; but, having a larger share of phosphates, it gives activity of muscle, especially the flesh of such fish as are themselves active, and may be adapted therefore to those whose labor requires great activity of muscle, and it is certainly good diet for work which requires study and judgment. (For an explanation of the principle that flesh of active animals develops activity, see Phil. Eat., page 84.) To enable us to judge of the amount and proportions of carbonaceous and nitrogenous elements necessary, I would refer to some practical experiments collated. (See Philosophy of Eating, pages 98–113.)

The English government has for many years carefully experimented on food for soldiers, and it is found that to keep them in good fighting trim, five ounces of nitrogenous and twenty ounces of carbonaceous food are required daily, and while in active service their rations always contain this amount of nourishment. The Dutch soldier has twenty-one ounces carbonates and five ounces nitrates while fighting, or preparing to fight; but in garrison, twenty ounces carbonates and three and one half ounces nitrates.

But our American commissaries seem not to have given sufficient attention to the subject, even to learn the difference between fat pork and lean beef. Accordingly, at one time our soldiers were obliged to march a whole day on twelve ounces of fat pork, which contains not a particle of food for muscles, and hard tack, which, being made of flour out of which is bolted a large part of its nitrates, could not in all that could be eaten contain one quarter of the nitrates necessary; while at another time the rations might consist of lean beef, which has in it little else than muscle-making food.

By all the facts that can be gathered from bills of fare of soldiers, sailors, prisoners, and other working men whose diet is accurately observed, it is ascertained that at the average temperature in which men work, and with the average activity, five ounces of carbonates and twenty-one ounces of nitrates are required; and in the staple articles of natural food, such as the meats, fat and lean together, and bread from unbolted grain, milk, eggs, &c., these necessary principles are found mixed in about the right proportions; and in eating them the appetite will be satisfied with the amount of food necessary to furnish these twenty-six ounces; but if he has set before him unnatural food, that is, food from which has been taken some of its principles, as butter, cheese, or beefsteak, fine flour, or sugar, his appetite will not direct him as to quantity. For example: He may eat of white bread and butter all the stomach will contain, and not be satisfied, because nature demands and the appetite craves more nutriment for the muscles and brain; or, on the other hand, he may eat of cheese, or beefsteak alone, twice as much as is needed for the muscles, while there is still a demand for carbon, which will not be satisfied till bread, or potatoes, or some other carbonaceous food is supplied. In either case he will eat too much; but if he have before him a variety of natural food, such as meats or grains or fish, and vegetables and fruits, he may indulge his appetite, especially in the early part of the day, to the fullest extent, without harm. Eating too much, then, comes of eating unnatural food. Why should not other animals, who have unrestrained access to their natural food, eat too much?

But how shall we guard against eating too much, while indulging in food not all in its natural condition? We have seen that some articles of food in common use, both in its natural and unnatural condition, contain too much of the carbonaceous and some too much of the nitrogenous elements, and we have seen by the tables of analysis, so often referred to, that it is easy to learn which articles contain the right proportions, and which contain an excess of either principle, and bearing in mind the proportions of each principle consumed, it is easy to adjust a dinner so as to supply the principles in right proportions.

If the meal consists of meats of average fatness, — more or less fat according to the temperature of the weather, — cooked by itself, and its juices saved, unbolted wheat bread, potatoes and other vegetables, with milk, and plain puddings from any grain in its natural state, and any good ripe fruits, we might eat as much as we desired of any or all the articles before us, without varying essentially the proportions of nitrates and carbonates, and without eating too much; or, if we have articles too nitrogenous — as beefsteak, or cheese, or beans, or peas — for dinner, it is only necessary to use with them articles like butter, fat meats, and starch or sugar, and vegetables, to supply the deficiency.

The difficulty is, that not knowing the constituents of food, we use together articles which are deficient in the same elements, as white bread and butter, pork and hard tack, sugar, butter, and flour, as in cake and pastry, &c. To remedy this evil, it is only necessary to refer to the tables of analysis. (See Philosophy of Eating, pages 121–126.) Assistance may also be obtained from the following table, which shows what quantity of articles of food in common use is required to get the five ounces of nitrates needed daily, and how much of carbonaceous food is had at the same time.

To get the requisite five ounces of nitrates requires, of

	Lbs.	Oz. Total.	Oz. Nitr.	Oz. Carb.	Pr. ct. Waste.	Pr. ct. Water.
Cheese, ...	0	8	5	3	0	0
Southern corn, .	1	2	5	6½	8	14
Beans, ...	1	8	5	10⅓	17	15
Peas, ...	1	9	5	10½	19	14
Barley, ...	2	5	5	22	16	14
Wheat, ...	2	7	5	21	3½	14
Oats, ...	2	0	5	19	15	13
Northern corn, .	2	9	5	24	5	14
Rye, ...	2	8	5	23	15	13
Rice, ...	5	0	5	50	4	13½
Buckwheat, . . .	4	0	5	35	3	14
Potatoes, ...	15	0	5	51	3	75
Sweet potato, .	20	0	5	65	1½	67
Carrots, ...	50	0	5	51	4½	87
Cabbage, ...	10	0	5	2	4	90
Turnips, ...	28	0	5	2	4	90
Parsnips, ...	25	0	5	25	9	82
Apples, &c., . .	5 to 10		5	5 to 10	5	86
Milk, ...	6	0	5	20	4	86
Beef, ...	4	0	5	45	5	44
Mutton, ...	4	0	5	64	4	44
Lamb, ...	4	0	5	35	3½	50
Veal, ...	4	0	5	28	4½	62

	Lbs. Oz. Total.	Oz. Nitr.	Oz. Carb.	Pr. ct. Waste.	Pr. ct. Water.
Pork, ...	5 8	5	110	1½	38
Lean beef, . .	1 4	5	0	7	70
Lean mutton, .	1 4	5	0	6½	70
Lean veal, . .	1 4	5	0	6	75
Lean pork, . .	1 5	5	10	3	60
Lean fish, . .	1 4	5	0	10	75
Butter, . . .	–	0	all	0	0
Lard, ...	–	0	"	0	0
Fat of all meats,	–	0	"	0	0
Starch, . . .	–	0	"	0	75
Sugar, . . .	–	0	"	0	75

Why is a Variety of Food necessary?

Besides the three staple principles for the supply of muscles, and animal heat, and the brain and nerves, included under the terms Nitrates, Carbonates, and Phosphates, other principles are needed and other conditions required to keep the digestive organs in perfect condition and the system in perfect working order.

1. We need food in amount or bulk sufficient to produce a proper degree of distention, else the digestive process cannot go on properly. The vegetarian eats on an average, perhaps, six pounds in a day, while of mixed food, of meat, unbolted bread, and vegetables, and fruits, the average may be four pounds. If, then, we should undertake to live on cheese alone, the stomach would collapse into one eighth of its natural size, and could not

secrete the necessary juices, or digest at all. With cheese, then, we must have vegetables or fruits, or other less concentrated food, for the purpose of distention; and the same remark applies to meats, beans, peas, &c., but to a less extent.

2. We must have also waste, which is the natural stimulant to produce the healthy action of all the digestive organs. If, then, we ate only cheese, or white bread and butter, or confectionery, or pastry, we should soon die of constipation.

3. The acids and juices provided in fruits and succulent vegetables are needed also every day, but more in warm weather than in cold, to eliminate from the system effete matter; and all nations, civilized or savage, make use of them: and if they are not had, the liver becomes engorged, the brain and the whole system becomes inactive, and, after a while, the skin breaks out in sores, and that degenerate condition or disease supervenes which is denominated scurvy, to which soldiers and sailors who are deprived of them are subject, and of which so many are known to die. (See Philosophy of Eating, pages 262–265.)

4. Food, to be well digested and assimilated, must be adapted to the taste of each individual; and a dinner made up of the necessary elements, but of articles against which we have an antipathy, or so cooked as to offend the taste, will not be digested at all, but will be rejected by the stomach, even while the system requires nourishment. (See Philosophy of Eating, pages 213–218, 306–311.)

With these considerations in mind, let us examine the foregoing table with a view to a more practical application to the every-day wants of the laboring man.

What Combination of Food will meet the daily Requirements of the Laboring Man?

The daily requirements are five ounces of solid nitrates for the muscles, twenty to twenty-two ounces of carbonates for animal heat, two or three per cent. of phosphates for bones and for nervous power, with waste and water to give it bulk, and acids to eliminate effete matter from the blood through the liver; and this food must be so prepared and cooked as to be eaten with a relish, and not be too easily digested.

By the foregoing table we see where we can get the five ounces of nitrogenous food, which is the first daily requisite for the laboring man, and we see that in the articles of food which come unchanged from Nature's storehouse, we have at the same time a part of all the other requisites, some containing too many for the ordinary demands of the system, and some not sufficient, making a variety of food necessary; and we have seen also that the natural appetite and taste directs to the use of such articles of natural food at the same meal as will supply all the demands of the system.

If, then, we had before us every variety of natural food, and nothing else, we might follow our inclinations to the fullest extent of our capacity without suffering evil consequences; but perverted as are our tastes and appetites by the constant use of butter, sugar, starch, and lard, which are separated from their food for muscles, nerves, and brains, our appetites and tastes are not a true guide, and we form a habit of taking too much carbonaceous food, with consequences such as are elsewhere described.

Under these circumstances, it becomes us to put our appetites under the guardianship of reason and common sense. And after all the mystery and darkness in which, in our ignorance, we have permitted this subject to be enshrouded, it is not a complicated question involving great mental power to comprehend, or memory to retain its principles. On the other hand, it is very simple, easily understood, and easily remembered.

Articles of Food in common Use containing an Excess of Nitrogenous Matter.

These are very few, and may all be embraced in the following articles: Cheese, southern corn, beans, peas, lean meats, fish, green vegetables, and fruits; and these require more or less food containing carbon in excess, as may be seen by the degree of deficiency noted in the preceding table; and all we have to do is to supply the deficiency with the articles containing an excess of carbon, as shown also in the table — only remembering that we require about twenty ounces carbonaceous food to five ounces nitrogenous.

Articles of Food in common Use containing an Excess of Carbonaceous Matter.

These consist of fats and oils, including butter, and of starch and sugar; and the articles of natural food in common use containing an excess of either of these principles are rice, buckwheat, potatoes, sweet potatoes, carrots, beets, and the meats of all domestic animals, as they are usually fattened for the market, and some species of fish used in northern regions. But the articles from which we derive most of our excess of heating food are the unnatural articles, — butter, sugar, lard, superfine flour (flour only containing anything but heating food, and that only a little), and in some places fat pork.

With these data before us, it requires but little study to understand what articles of food are to be used at the same meal, and what combination of articles should be avoided. It would be folly to undertake to live on cheese, or beans, or peas, or lean meat, or fish alone, or all of them combined. We should lose our fat, and become cold and die, for want of natural warmth of blood. It is equal folly to try to live on butter, sugar, fine flour, or lard, or all combined, as in pastry, cake, &c. Animals submitted to the experiment of such a combination alone, have died in from thirty to forty days; and probably three fourths of all the deaths recorded in our bills of mortality are the results of over-heated blood, and consequent inflammations and diseases induced by the excess of carbonaceous food on the organs and functions, rendered weak, and their recuperative power lost or greatly impaired, for want of the strength-giving nitrates and phosphates required, as has been elsewhere explained. (See Philosophy of Eating, pages 16, 17.)

How few and simple, then, are the requirements necessary so to combine the principles of food that are within the reach of all industrious families in this country at least, as to insure at the same time economy, the pleasures of eating, health, long life, and usefulness; and to all but the most perverse and ungrateful, cheerfulness, and domestic peace and happiness! I venture the assertion that with one quarter of the time, and without any of the expense that is devoted to the silly and ridiculous foibles made necessary by the demand of fashion, these blessings might be secured to all intelligent families; and instead of losing, as they now do, one half of their children before they come to maturity, and finding most of the other half feeble, sickly, and worthless, except, perhaps, a very few who might die from casualties and from diseases inherited from a degenerate ancestry, their sons would "be as plants grown up in their youth," and their daughters "as corner-stones, polished after the similitude of a palace."

THE ECONOMY OF TAKING FOOD IN NATURAL PROPORTIONS.

By something like a telegraphic arrangement the stomach is kept informed of the wants of every organ and function; and, through the appetite, a demand is made for nitrates for muscular strength, or carbonates for animal heat, or phosphates for bones, and nerves, and brain, until all are supplied. And if we take food in its natural state, so as to supply all these demands at the same time, the appetite is satisfied without waste material. For example, take unbolted wheat bread and milk, containing, as they both do, a due proportion of elements for muscle, animal heat, and brains. The appetite is satisfied when just enough food is taken to supply the ten ounces of carbonates and two and a half ounces of nitrates, for twelve hours' supply. But suppose we take, instead, white flour bread and butter. When we have taken the ten ounces of carbonates which the system requires for the meal, we have received less than one quarter of the necessary nitrates and phosphates, and until these principles are supplied the appetite demands more food; and if we attempt to satisfy these demands by the same food, we must take four times as much of carbonates as are needed, and the surplus, not being wanted, after embarrassing the system for a time, is finally thrown off into the vault. And thus, by our daily habit of using, with articles already having their natural proportion of carbonates, butter, sugar, and fine flour, as we do in cakes, pastry, confectionery, sweet sauces, &c., we waste three quarters of all these expensive articles.

With less than half the expense that is thus wasted on these articles, to say nothing of the doctor's bills and loss of time occasioned by inflammatory diseases, we might purchase all the choice fruits, and vegetables, and meats necessary to give us the highest gustatory pleasures of which we are capable ; and, at the same time, save doctor's bills and loss of time from sickness. On natural food, therefore, judiciously selected, a family can be raised, in the full enjoyment of robust health, and substantial, enduring happiness, for less than half the cost of trying to keep alive our feeble, pale-faced, sickly children on white bread and butter, pies, cakes, and candy.

NATURAL FOOD AFFORDS THE HIGHEST GUSTATORY ENJOYMENT.

THAT is certainly a beautiful provision of our heavenly Father, by which perfect happiness is made to consist in perfect obedience to his laws; and this pertains to every department of our nature, moral and physical. Indeed, there can be no real, unalloyed enjoyment but in perfect obedience to moral, mental, physiological, or physical law. It may be true in dietetics, as it is in morals, that "no man liveth and sinneth not," and therefore no man enjoys perfect, unalloyed pleasures in eating; but in the one case, as in the other, he enjoys most who most nearly obeys the laws of his nature.

Every article of natural food is provided with its own particular flavor, or *osmazome*, which distinguishes it from every other article; and this *osmazome* is most perfectly developed just when it is so prepared as to be best adapted to furnish us wholesome nourishment. Beefsteak has its most agreeable flavor developed with just the amount of cooking that best fits it for digestion. And this is true of all meats and vegetables; while the peach, and other fruits which need no cooking, have their most agreeable flavor developed without cooking, and, when fully ripe, the slightest amount of cooking diminishes their flavor, as any extra cooking or re-cooking of meats and vegetables diminishes their flavor, and renders them less wholesome. (For a full explanation of this beautiful principle, see Philosophy of Eating, pages 213–218, 306, 311.)

This principle, *osmazome*, seems to be imparted for no other purpose than to make food agreeable, and give us gustatory pleasure. And of course our natural tastes are made to harmonize with these natural flavors, so as to enable us to appreciate and enjoy them; and, until they are perverted, we do enjoy them — just as all other pleasures of the senses afford pleasure unalloyed till perverted.

A child who has never tasted of pies, cakes, candy, or any other unnatural food, will much prefer wheat bread and milk, or fruit, to any of them. This I have seen in a grandson four years old, who had eaten nothing but milk, unbolted meal bread, fruits, and other natural food, and who, in a large party of little ones, all eating cakes and confectionery, could not be induced to eat a thing, till he found an apple, which he recognized as natural food. The inference, then, that butter and sugar must be good, because children love them, is fallacious. Their natural love is for butter and sugar as they are found in milk and fruits, in their natural combinations with other necessary elements.

The first time sugar or butter is given to a child the sensation is such as to produce a shudder, and the little victim clearly indicates a disapprobation of such concentrated sapidity; but he so soon yields to his fate that parents come to think his love for these things is natural. The taste is generally tampered with in the first hour of life, by the sugar and water which its thoughtful nurse administers lest the poor thing might starve before Nature gets ready to provide for it; and then, for the hickups which this unnatural feeding is sure to produce, it must have pure sugar; and thus the taste is perverted in the first week of its life, and then the first solid food that is put into its mouth is, probably, white bread, spread, perhaps, with butter.

No, no; Nature is not so inconsistent as to give us a natural taste for unnatural food. Nothing, to my mind, can be clearer than that the responsibility of the love of concentrated carbonaceous food, which undoubtedly causes, directly or indirectly, three fourths of all the sickness, suffering, and death of our children, rests on parents. And yet how hard it is to convince them that what their mothers did for them, and what they lived through, can be wrong.

In vain you remind them of their less hardy brothers and sisters, who have long since been laid in the grave from inflammations and other diseases induced by heating food. In vain you show them the reasonableness of obeying Nature's laws, and the fact that animals who do obey them enjoy health, and lose none of their offspring. Their only answer is, "I feed my child as my mother fed me. I did very well. I guess the little sugar, and cake, and white bread and butter which I give won't hurt them." But, I thank God, *there are those* who have sense enough to see the folly of such persistence in wrong, and who, giving reason and common sense control over silly prejudices, pursue the right as soon as they learn it. Such will have the happiness to see their brains transmitted to healthy and useful children, while those whose only rule is to do as their mothers did before them will transmit a race more silly, feeble, and degenerate than themselves (for the evil effects of disobedience accumulate from generation to generation), and will see them living a life of struggle with disease and suffering, or will prematurely bury them, murmuring, perhaps, at the cruelty of their fate.

Suppose a mother, in ordinary health, having a healthy husband, should always live on natural food, or, at least, should commence, seven or eight months before her child is born, and allow nothing to pass her lips but food containing all the elements that nature has furnished in it, and should take no elements in liquids but such as Nature furnishes in the juices of fruits, vegetables, milk, and pure water, and continue that course, without exception, till the child is old enough to be weaned; — having all the materials for making a perfect child, just as they are naturally provided, will Nature fail to use these materials, so as to leave any organ or function defective? Having lime, silex, potash, and insoluble phosphates for the bones and teeth, with no foreign elements to interfere with the process of forming them, perfect teeth will surely be formed. Having nitrogenous elements for muscles and solid tissues, soluble phosphates and other materials for the brain and nerves, carbon and hydrogen for adipose matter and to furnish animal heat, and all these elements and principles in the combinations and proportions which she herself has adjusted, Nature cannot fail to furnish a child perfect in all its parts and functions.

Then, supposing it continues to be furnished with natural food and drinks, allowing no foreign elements to enter the system, and conforming to other necessary requirements as to pure air, cleanliness, exercise, comfortable temperature, protection, &c., when can the organs or functions begin to be imperfect, or to become diseased? Indeed, if he should not, in all respects, conform to laws of his being, his constitution, being kept in order by natural food, will have recuperative power to ward off or overcome the evil effects, and health, nevertheless, be continued or restored. Then, again, with recuperative powers, derived from conforming to Nature's laws, and living on natural food, diseases from external causes, as small-pox, measles, &c., could all be controlled, and made harmless. Surely, then, it is a sin and a shame, as well as a misfortune, to have feeble, half-developed, sickly children; and, instead of murmuring at the Providence that removes them from us, we should repent, in dust and ashes, that, by our neglect of the clearly-revealed laws of Nature, it becomes a merciful necessity to remove them from the evil to come; and if too late, for benefit to ourselves and our children, to do works meet for repentance, we should cease not to teach the young the laws of life and health, and "to warn every one, night and day, with tears," to escape the punishment which has been inflicted on us for our transgressions. But we shall meet a class of cases harder to reach than those who have suffered the loss of health and the loss of children.

Those who live and seem to enjoy Health in spite of wrong Habits of living.

An old toper, who has kept his copper hot with whiskey or rum for half a century, and who has outlived all his drinking companions by scores of years, cannot see that he lives because he is too tough to be killed by that which has killed all his old toper friends, but very likely thinks he should have been dead long ago but for the preserving power of alcohol.

An excellent old lady of seventy-five years, who had taken green tea from her youth, till by the tannin it contained her skin had been dried and tanned into the resemblance of what indeed it really was, dark-brown leather, said to a friend, in sober earnest, "There will probably be very few more old people in Boston, for everybody is leaving off drinking green tea."

After Carnaro lived fifty-eight years on twelve ounces of solid food and fourteen ounces of light wines each day, containing a mere trifle of alcohol, Professor Lewes (himself a drinker of alcohol), "wonders that intelligent men, in view of such a fact, can doubt that alcohol is nutritious."

I have tried in vain to persuade a young mother, who has inherited a good constitution, and who is one of six children, all but two of whom lived to maturity, the remaining four, however, being subject to dyspepsia, neuralgia, colics, and all the other sufferings induced by too heating food, to bring up her child in obedience to Nature's laws, trying to show her that the chances of its living to grow up will be doubled, and her exemption from suffering vastly greater, as it will be less liable to sickness, and have greater recuperative power to overcome it; but she says she is willing to trust her child with the same treatment that she herself had, and lived through, and so in the first winter of life the top of its lungs are exposed by low-necked dresses, and it is fed with sugar, cakes, white bread and butter, &c., and now, as it has lived through the winter and spring without lung fever, — as I told her it might not, — she is fully confirmed that she is right, and will probably go on risking its life further and further till, unless it proves tougher than the majority of children, some inflammatory disease will take it from them; and even then it is hardly probable she will be convinced of her responsibility in the case. And thus it is now, as in the times of Ecclesiastes the Preacher, "Because sentence against an evil work is not executed speedily, therefore the heart of the sons of men is fully set in them to do evil."

FOOD FOR SEDENTARY PEOPLE.

By experiments made on five hundred prisoners, in five jails in Scotland, it was found that the least amount of food that would keep men up to their standard weight while sitting still in a moderate temperature, was four ounces of solid nitrogenous food and thirteen ounces of carbonaceous. (See Philosophy of Eating, page 98.) And we see in another chapter that soldiers in active service, and laboring men, require from twenty to twenty-three ounces of carbonates and five ounces of nitrates.

By these data we can estimate the amount of these principles required in different degrees of exercise, but we must also consider the difference in quality of food adapted to different conditions. Laboring men require more of such nitrogenous food as gives most fibre and strength of muscle, as the flesh of active animals, cheese, beans, peas, &c., which contain fibrine and casein, which make fibrine for the muscles; while sedentary men require more of gluten and albumen, which are found in fish, eggs, grain, &c. Then, again, the carbonates which are adapted to sedentary life are sugar and starch, rather than most of the fat of meats, and they need more of acids to eliminate effete matter from the liver, which accumulates for want of activity. They need, also, more waste material, to keep the bowels in action, and therefore require, besides the grains in their natural state, more vegetables and fruits, which furnish waste as well as acids; and these waste and acid principles are needed more in spring than at any other time, especially the acid fruits. Not that that is Nature's arrangement, or that these requirements would be needed if we lived in winter as we should; but sedentary people spend most of their time in winter in a warm atmosphere, and need, therefore, vegetables and fruits almost as much as in summer; but not having them, and eating more of the fatty materials which produce this state of things, the liver becomes engorged with effete matter, which vegetable food alone is adapted to remove.

This can be tolerated in winter, when the system has more physical energy, especially if a part of the time is spent in the open air. But when warm weather comes on, and the system becomes dormant, the liver, partaking of the general inactivity, cannot perform the extra duties of disgorging matter thus accumulated, and jaundice, and other bilious difficulties ensue. In such cases medicines which act directly on the liver may afford temporary relief; but Nature's sovereign remedy is found in the juices of fruits and vegetables.

Sedentary people not only need different kinds of food from active laborers, but they require it differently cooked. Active men can live and thrive on salted and boiled meats, as I have before explained, out of which have been taken the soluble phosphates and the albumen, because they retain the elements which give strength to bones and muscles; but these last elements are essential to sedentary men, as are also the sugar, albumen, and soluble phosphates of vegetables, which are lost in soaking and boiling in water, unless the water in which they are boiled or soaked is retained and used as gravy or soup.

Active men, having also good digestive powers, can dispose of food out of which is taken, by salting, or soaking or boiling, the osmazome, or flavor, which so essentially assists in the digestion of food; but those who have little out-of-door exercise, and require less food, having less powers of digestion, need the aid of all these flavors, and every other auxiliary to digestion. They should, therefore, have all their food so cooked as to retain every element and every quality which Nature has provided in it, so as to make it most agreeable to the taste, and most digestible.

Flavor, which is essential to good Digestion, is volatile, and may be lost in cooking.

That principle which gives relish to food, and which distinguishes one article from another, called *osmazome*, I have elsewhere explained (see Philosophy of Eating, pages 307–310), and I propose here only to show how it can be preserved in cooking.

Go into any house where meats and vegetables are being cooked in the open air in the basement, and you find the air filled with the combined flavor of every article. Of course all the flavor thus diffused is lost for the purpose for which Nature intended it, and the food is rendered insipid to the extent to which it is thus diffused, and to the same extent it becomes indigestible. This is proved by the fact adverted to (Philosophy of Eating, page 214), where good meat was boiled in the open air till all its osmazome was removed, but which retained all other essential elements; and the stomach of the dog, which was allowed no other food, so rejected it that, rather than eat it, he would have died of starvation.

All meats and vegetables should therefore be cooked by a process which not only saves the soluble nitrates, phosphates, and carbonates, as before stated, but also the osmazome; and for that purpose, the steamer invented by Zimmermann, and improved by Duncklee, is an admirable arrangement, saving, as it does, all the flavor, and condensing it in the water at the bottom, so that the smell is not perceptible in the house or kitchen in which it is cooked, and so that it may all be returned to the meats or vegetables, vastly improving their flavor and digestibility.

The flavor of soups may also be greatly improved by putting together every article to be used, first soaking them in cold water, and using that water only in the steamer, then steaming them gently, so as not to allow the steam to escape, and serving all the liquid that remains, diluted more or less to suit the taste. Soup thus made, with a variety of vegetables, and one kind of meat not before cooked, is to an unperverted taste delicious, without the addition of a single condiment except a little salt, (and the taste may be trained to relish soup and other food without salt; but there is no evidence that a little is injurious. Cattle that have access to salt eat all they want without injury.) Of course its flavor may be varied to suit the tastes of the family, by using such vegetables as are most agreeable, and by avoiding any article known to be offensive to any.

Roast meats may also be greatly improved by first steaming them for a short time with the vegetables to be used, and saving the water, to be used with the drippings of the meat for gravy, instead of the vile stuff made of flour and butter and spices, which is usually served for gravy.

Only one kind of meat should ever be cooked in the same steamer or roaster at the same time; otherwise, by mixing the flavors, all meats taste alike, and we get no variety. For this reason, hotel life soon becomes tiresome, and the food loathsome. All the meats being cooked in the same oven, and served with the same gravy, you may call for beef, pork, veal, mutton, or chicken, but cannot tell by the taste which you get.

For other important considerations pertaining to the adaptation of food to our circumstances, and the deleterious influences of all products of decomposition and chemical changes, as vinegar, alcohol, phosphates, iron, &c., and all other substances not prepared in Nature's laboratory, see Philosophy of Eating, under their respective heads.

FOOD FOR WINTER.

THAT carbonaceous food furnishes animal heat is clearly proved, and that, therefore, we need more starch, or fat, to keep us warm in winter, just as we need more coal and wood to warm our apartments, there is no doubt. Some hypercritical professor, who rides theoretical physiology as a hobby, may again object to the comparison, unless I fully explain the difference between combustion of fuel and the vital process by which animal heat is produced; but if I am able so to explain to common-sense minds the use of carbonaceous food, as to enable them to obtain its benefits and avoid its evils, I care very little for cavilling criticism. I have already explained the fact that fats and oils, having in them no water, contain two and one half times more carbon than starch and sugar, that contain a large per cent. of water. Fats and oils, therefore, are adapted to cold weather, when large supplies of heat are needed; and accordingly Nature furnishes this principle in cold climates, in the adipose covering of the flesh of seals, whales, and other animals which need it for their own protection from the cold, and also in the corn and grains, which contain oil as well as starch in proportion to the cold of the climate in which it grows. (See plates of Northern and Southern corn in

Philosophy of Eating, page 25.) So that the Greenlander may have his excessive demand for heat supplied by the excessive fatness of the seals and bears of that region, and the Canadian can be supplied by the oil and starch of his corn, either directly in his corn cakes, or indirectly in the fat which they furnish to his pigs and cattle.

People who live in the open air in cold climates are not in danger of eating too much carbonaceous food, even the gallon of whale oil, or twelve pounds of candles, which an Esquimaux woman is said to eat in a day, being only enough to keep up the necessary heat. But they who live in warm houses, and seldom go out in the cold, may and generally do eat too much carbonaceous food; and not having in winter so much of the counteracting influence of fruits and succulent vegetables, suffer even more from that cause than in summer.

Why is it that we suffer more from inflammatory diseases, especially of the throat, air passages and lungs, in winter than in summer? Eating, as we do in winter, more fat meat, buttered cakes, buckwheats, &c., with less of fruits and vegetables, and spending most of our time in warm rooms, we keep up that heated condition of the system which predisposes it to inflammations, and exposing, as we do, perhaps, for twenty-three out of the twenty-four hours, the nasal organs, air passages and lungs, to a warm and relaxing atmosphere, and then for one hour, perhaps, exposing them to air below the freezing point, and perhaps at zero, the vessels of the mucous membranes are first expanded and filled with blood, and then suddenly contracted and the blood expelled.

This naturally causes inflammation of the parts thus exposed, rather than other parts not thus exposed, and thus in winter we have catarrh, sore throat, bronchitis, lung fevers, &c., unless perchance we get a chill on some muscles or other organs by exposure to currents of air or damp clothing; then we may have, instead, rheumatism or gout, or some other disease to which we may be predisposed.

Nature evidently made provision in each climate for us to live mostly in the open air; for we find that the starch in grains and seeds, and the proportion of fat in all animals, compared with the muscle-making elements, are furnished in proportion to the average amount of cold for the year of the climate in which the animals or grains grow or live. For example: The weight of wheat is mostly made up of starch and gluten; and hundreds of analyses have been made to ascertain their relative proportions in different climates of Europe, and it is found to vary from the cold northern states of Scotland and Northern Russia, from ten per cent. of gluten in these northern climates to thirty-five per cent. in Italy and Turkey and the more southern climates, the remainder being mostly starch. And the same fact has been shown by comparing the wheat of Canada with that of Georgia and Alabama in this country. And to show that this is not an accidental circumstance, wheat from Canada has been sown and raised in Georgia, and the first year it will produce nearly the amount of starch as the same kind in Canada; but if the product be again raised in Georgia, the next crop will contain less starch, and it will thus continue to diminish, if continuously raised, till its proportions are the same as Georgia wheat; and the change will be reversed by raising Georgia wheat in Canada; and the same effect is produced by the same process on corn and other grain. For those, therefore, who in this climate live mostly in warm houses, and spend but little time in open air, and for warm weather, bread from Southern corn and Southern wheat is much more wholesome than from Northern corn or wheat.

We cannot of course always live in the open air in winter, or avoid sudden changes of temperature, and the important practical question is, How can we avoid the evils produced by these changes? Of bathing, friction, muscular exercise, as giving the system recuperative power, and power to resist the effects of changes, I have elsewhere written. (See Philosophy of Eating, under their respective heads.)

CHRONIC DISEASES CURED BY DIET.

In another chapter I have shown that extra carbonaceous food, by keeping up the heat of the blood above its natural temperature, predisposes the whole system to fevers and inflammations, and renders these fevers and inflammations less easily cured, just as exposure of wood and other combustible substances to heat renders them liable to combustion, and makes it more difficult to subdue the flames if once commenced.

Extra carbonaceous food, then, is the predisposing cause of catarrhs, sore throats, lung fevers, and inflammations generally. The exciting cause is change of temperature, producing undue contraction and expansion of blood vessels; but if there is sufficient recuperative power in the system, these diseases will be prevented or immediately thrown off.

Accordingly we find that the same exposure which will produce disease in one person will be entirely harmless in another; and some facts have recently come to light which go to corroborate the idea that those who take no extra carbonaceous food have power not only to resist the encroachments of disease, but have recuperative powers that produce wonderful effects in the cure of disease: so that, living according to Nature's laws, we may not only hope to be exempt from new diseases, but may also get rid of chronic diseases and infirmities of even twenty-five years' standing.

My attention was first called to this fact by the statement of Banting, the fat Englishman, who reduced his weight by abstaining from carbonaceous, and eating freely of nitrogenous and phosphatic food, that while living on this diet, a hernia, for which he had worn a truss for many years, was almost entirely cured; and during the last year a case has come under my observation still more remarkable. A gentleman who has been obliged to wear a truss for inguinal hernia for nearly twenty-five years, and who is now sixty-four years old, having for the last two years eaten no extra carbonaceous food, has been gradually recovering from the hernia, and now for some months has left off his truss entirely. At first these cures seemed to me almost miraculous; at least I could see no connection between the cause and effect; but on reflection, I am convinced that the explanation is this: Hernia is caused by want of tone and consequent relaxation of the abdominal muscles, occasioned, perhaps, generally by want of sufficient nitrogenous food. The tendons are not drawn together sufficiently taut at the ring to retain perfectly the flowing and slippery intestines, and they pass through; but by leaving off extra carbonates, and taking instead the nitrogenous food, which gives strength to muscles, their tone is restored, the tendons are drawn taut, and the bowels are retained.

The following case of family idiosyncrasy I think gives some light on the influence of nitrogenous food on the muscular tissues: A few years since, a physician in Boston, in a good but not harassing practice, became so affected by disease of the heart that for a long time — I think a year — he could not attend to business, and at times was brought apparently to the point of death. He travelled from city to city, consulting all the most eminent physicians in the country, especially such as made heart disease a specialty. They all agreed that his case was anomalous; and inasmuch as his father and one brother had died of a similar disease, they naturally supposed his would prove fatal also. But he recovered, and is now enjoying good health and engaged in active practice.

Knowing that he was an extravagant eater of cheese, — the most concentrated nitrogenous food in the catalogue (see Philosophy of Eating, page 122), — and seeing the extraordinary effects of such food in the cases just referred to, and, therefore, suspecting that cheese might have had something to do with the case, I called on him, and obtained the following facts: —

His father and his brother, as well as himself, were all extravagant eaters of cheese; eating it at all times in the day, and in great quantities; and they had, of course, great powers of digestion: for a stomach that can digest cheese in half-pound quantities can digest anything. And the old gentleman died at eighty-four, of what was considered organic disease of the heart, retaining his digestive powers to the last. The brother died comparatively young, with similar symptoms; and the doctor, after struggling for a long time with similar symptoms, seemed to be approaching a similar end, when he gave up cheese for a time, and soon began to recover. Since then, for two or three years, having eaten less than half his former quantity of cheese, he seems perfectly well.

The doctor's case was not, of course, organic disease, and my diagnosis of the three cases is this: All eating probably two or three times more nitrogenous and phosphatic food than was necessary to supply the requisite muscular and nervous power, and, as in the cases referred to, where the right proportions of this kind of food gave new tone to the abdominal muscles, and enabled them to overcome a hernia and cure it, so in their cases, excess of the same food produced an excessive tone and tension to the muscular system, and the heart, being a muscular organ, the action of which must be regular and not excessive, to perform its functions properly, that was the organ on which this excess of tone and tension most clearly manifested itself, and the symptoms were precisely such as might have been expected under such circumstances.

The circulation was very rapid, and the pulse very full and irregular, and at times, for eighteen hours without ceasing, the heart would beat with such force as to jar the bed on which the doctor lay, and then suddenly, as if exhausted, would calm down as if to rest.

With recuperative powers such as is induced by such food and such powers of digestion, Nature holds out wonderfully, and for a whole year she was able to grapple with the difficulty, till relief finally came by removing the cause; and now, if he will allow himself to take no more nitrogenous food than is necessary, say five ounces in a day, his chances of life are as good as those of any other man in the same circumstances in other respects.

His brother, continuing his extra nitrogenous diet to the last, and, having less recuperative power, perhaps, succumbed to the first attack in two or three weeks. His father, having extraordinary vital energy, endured the strain of extra nervous and muscular power to a good old age, but, continuing his extraordinary diet to the last, he yielded also to the first attack.

But other cases show more directly the recuperative effect of natural food. A gentleman of scrofulous tendencies, who had had for eight or ten years an open abscess, was induced, for the improvement of his general health, to abstain from extra carbon, and take food rich in nitrogen and phosphorus, and almost immediately the abscess began to heal, and in a few weeks it ceased to discharge, and this without any local application to it.

Another gentleman had a kind of gouty enlargement of the great toe joints, which had become chronic, and which required boots of extra width to enable him to walk. For improvement in general health, he also adopted natural food exclusively, and in a few months could wear narrow, genteel boots, without the least pain or inconvenience.

These three very suggestive cases have come under my observation within the last year; and among the large number who have already adopted practically "the Philosophy of Eating" (even now reckoned by hundreds), there are probably other cases that have not been brought to my notice.*

These cases, though not sufficient to establish an important theory, at least give us reason to hope for more benefit from living philosophically than I had dared to anticipate. They show at least that, to some extent, abstaining from extra carbonaceous food and using instead that which is nitrogenous and phosphatic, the system has increased power not only to resist the encroachments of diseases, but also to overcome and cure them.

* If any persons, who, on abstaining from extra carbonaceous food, may have experienced incidental benefit in regard to long standing or other infirmities or diseases, will report to me the facts in their cases, they may subserve the interests both of science and humanity.

FOOD FOR SUMMER.

In warm climates Nature provides starch and sugar for necessary animal heat, and fat and gluten and albumen for muscular power; while in cold climates fat and starch are the carbonates. Ripe fruits and green vegetables have mostly sugar for their carbonates, and gluten and albumen for their nitrates. Grains and seeds have mostly starch for carbonates, and gluten and albumen for their nitrates; and it is worthy of notice that while grain, especially corn growing in the Northern States and Canada, has a large share of oil, the corn of Southern states has not a sixth as much.

Animals, also, of northern climates, eating the grain that contains fattening oil, have much more adipose covering to their flesh than the same species in southern climates. These are clear intimations that sugar and starch are appropriate principles for furnishing animal heat in warm weather, and fat and starch in cold weather.

We also find a larger proportion of starch in wheat and corn (Southern corn having but half the starch in proportion to gluten as Northern corn), and, indeed, in all grains in northern climates. (See plate of Northern and Southern corn in Philosophy of Eating, page 25.) We find, also, that the warmer the climate the greater the abundance of succulent vegetables and fruits, whose carbonates consist almost entirely of sugar. And from all these facts we are shown that vegetables, grains, and fruits are intended for warm weather, and that meats, especially fat meats, are better adapted to cold weather. Fish, however, of every climate, furnishes appropriate food for that climate; those of northern waters being fatter than those of southern.

A little reflection on these data will suggest a bill of fare for warm weather, consisting of the grains in their natural state, — avoiding Northern corn and wheat, — vegetables, fruits and berries, as they come along, the most succulent being furnished in the warmest part of the season, with lean meats and fish, and only enough of butter or fat to make them palatable, avoiding, especially, stimulating condiments and concentrated combinations of heating food, as pastry, cakes, flour puddings, white bread and butter, &c., these carbonaceous articles of food being undoubtedly a predisposing cause of the dysenteries, dyspepsias, liver and bowel complaints, that are so prevalent in warm weather.

And it is not an argument against this theory that nursing children are as liable to these diseases as others; for, according to the doctrine I have endeavored to establish, the influence of carbonaceous food is the same on the nursing child, through the mother, as on the weaned child directly. Nor is it an argument against the free use of fruits and vegetables, that, if taken only occasionally, and in excess, they produce or excite these very diseases; for it is true in this case, as in every other, that that which in regular use and appropriate quantities is wholesome, in irregular use and in excess is the source of suffering and disease. Besides, if children were constantly supplied with fresh and wholesome fruits and vegetables, they would never eat them in excess. (For further development of these principles, see Philosophy of Eating, page 139, also the chapter on Dyspepsia.)

PREVENTION AND CURE OF DYSPEPSIA.

THE grand port of entry for the human system is the stomach, and the senses of taste and smell are placed, as sentinels, to guard its portals; and, if not tampered with and demoralized, they would not, under any pretence, allow a particle of matter, solid or liquid, to enter it, except food as organized and prepared in Nature's own laboratory, and drinks composed of milk, the juices of fruits and plants, and pure water; and these would only be admitted as they are needed to supply the necessary elements as fast as they are used up and cast off from the system.

All animals in their natural state range at large in the sphere assigned them, and have access to everything, good and bad; but their appetites and tastes, as sentinels and guardian angels, allow not a particle that would be injurious to enter the stomach. Though there might be found in the same field, and even in the same plant, the natural food and the deadly poison, they are directed, with unerring certainty, to take such food as contains the elements required to keep them in health, and to reject everything that would be injurious. Having, therefore, all that is requisite to keep the stomach and digestive organs in health, and nothing to disturb their secretions and functions, they never have dyspepsia, or any other disease, except such as are induced by accident.

Does any one doubt that man would be as perfectly exempt from dyspepsia, and, indeed, from all other diseases, if he lived as entirely on natural food, and obeyed as perfectly all the laws of his nature? To believe otherwise is to believe that our Maker has taken less care of his most perfect work than of his inferior productions. Do you say that man has less power to discriminate between the good and the bad because his senses of smell and taste are less acute? That may be true; but are not his intellect and reason more than an equivalent for any deficiency in his animal senses? Our senses of smell and taste are, however, sufficiently acute to guide us, if unperverted by the use of food out of which has been taken some of its essential elements, and by poisonous articles. And, as it is, they are faithful sentinels still, as far as they are allowed to be, and admit no food in its natural condition but at the right time and in right quantities; so that, in regard to the grains, meats, milk, vegetables, and fruits, in their natural state, if we ate nothing else, we might eat as much of them as the appetite demanded, without injury.

But a faithful sentinel might admit to the garrison one who might prove to be the vilest traitor or spy; and though, at first, he might be suspicious of him, might, after a while, come to like him, and treat him with kindness, if, at first, he had been ordered to admit him by a superior officer; — so these sentinels of the stomach admit, and come to have confidence in, and even ardently love, not only butter, sugar, starch, fat, and other articles which are injurious, in that unnatural, concentrated state in which we use them, but even the vilest weeds and compounds containing the most poisonous principles, as tobacco, alcoholic drinks, opium, hashish, &c. Under these circumstances, it may be questioned whether, with these perverted appetites and tastes, it is possible to return to natural food alone, so as to bring back the system to its normal condition, and make it exempt from the diseases and suffering to which it is thus made liable.

Whether or not it is possible to restore a degenerate and diseased body to a state of perfect health, one thing is encouraging: — we find, by the testimony of all who resolve to live as nearly right as possible, that they succeed in improving their condition far beyond their expectations, and that just in proportion as they approximate to Nature's standard is their approximation to health, as also to the enjoyments of eating; and in just the proportion as they eat natural food, properly cooked, and allow nothing else to enter the stomach, are they free from dyspepsia, and the thousand and one pains and ills that are connected with it.

Animals in their natural state never suffer from dyspepsia, because, from the day of their birth till the day of their death, being left free to follow their natural appetites and tastes, they never take into their stomachs a particle of matter, solid or liquid, but natural food and pure water; but the appetites and tastes of children are not left unperverted for a single day,— "they go astray as soon as they be born,"—and that child is a lucky exception who escapes unnatural food for the first six hours of life: as if Nature was so at fault as not to provide nourishment as soon as it is needed. As a natural consequence, the symptoms of dyspepsia, such as flatulence, colic, &c., commence on the first day of life; and then come the catnip and camomile teas, to relieve the flatulence and pains induced by the sugar, which are sure to induce other pains worse and more enduring; and thus, on the first day of life is inaugurated, not only dyspepsia, but, at the same time, a system of treatment which perpetuates all manner of diseases and sufferings to the end of life, and which diminishes the average length of life from "threescore years and ten" to from thirty to thirty-three years. And the foundation for these evils is also laid during the period of nursing, and even before birth, as I have before explained, by the neglect of the mother to furnish elements for a perfect organization, and by furnishing, instead, elements which, not being needed, are injurious.

And having, in such culpable ignorance, laid the foundation, and inaugurated a system, and formed appetites for unnatural food, by which these diseases and sufferings are so early commenced, we, of course, follow on, thoughtlessly, in the way in which our parents have started us, in the use of heating food and deleterious drugs, till we inevitably fall a prey to the diseases which are thus induced and perpetuated. And, to every reflecting mind, the wonder is, not that so many are troubled with dyspepsia, but rather that any escape.

The Process of Digestion.

The most important agents in the process of digestion are the juices of the mouth, the stomach, the liver, and pancreas — the gastric juice being the most important, the others being only auxiliary. These juices are changed day by day, in certain qualities, so as to be adapted to the digestion of different kinds of food, and, like muscles which have regular duties to perform, have power given them according to the duties required. If we live on food requiring little power of digestion, like rice, fine flour, fresh fish, soups, &c., the powers of digestion will, after a while, become so enfeebled that, if suddenly we take solid meat, cheese, &c., suitable juices not being, at first, furnished, indigestion, or temporary dyspepsia, follows; but continue the use of these articles, and the appropriate juices will be furnished, and the powers of digestion will rally and perform the task assigned them. It is a mistake to suppose that the most digestible food is best for those who are predisposed to dyspepsia; on the other hand, the powers of the stomach are capable of cultivation, and become strong or weak according to the regular work imposed on them to do, just as the muscles become strong or weak as they are or are not actively used. But in the one case, as in the other, strength can be imparted only by regular and gradually increasing exercise. Perhaps, for example, there is not one stomach in twenty which, after a lengthy abstinence from it, could readily digest cheese; and yet there is not one stomach in a thousand that could not be made to digest it readily, by beginning its use in small quantities early in the day, and increasing the quantity daily; and thus we may teach the stomach, as we may teach the muscles, to perform any reasonable task regularly imposed on it. This is an important consideration, both as a means of preventing and curing dyspepsia.

Another important consideration relates to the principle which gives relish to food, called *osmazome* — a principle without which the digestive juices are not secreted, and without which digestion cannot go on at all. This is proved by the experiment already referred to, in which the dog, shut up with meat having all its elements preserved but the flavor, would not eat it, because it could not be digested, although he was starving. Our own experience also shows us how much our digestion depends on the relish with which it is taken. And we are thus taught that it is our bounden duty to enjoy eating as it is our duty to enjoy life. But we find in the one case, as in the other, that true enjoyment comes only in connection with obedience to the laws of our being; so that they enjoy most who only study to know what is duty, while they enjoy least who only seek after enjoyment in eating, and most assiduously inquire what can be had that is good to eat.

So also in the one case, as in the other, the pleasures

which we do enjoy, in the unnatural excitements of excess, are fraught with evil consequences, and produce subsequent reaction, depression, exhaustion, or suffering — as, in the other case, the pleasures derived from the taste of sugar, butter, flour, and their combinations, give us, in just the proportion as their flavor is excessive and unnatural, subsequent gastric exhaustion, debility, disease, and pain.

To get, then, all the gustatory enjoyment we are capable of receiving, we have but to take, every day, the kind and variety of food best suited to the condition and duties of the body for that day — so kind is our heavenly Father, in providing that, in keeping his commandments, physical and moral, there is always great reward, and in thus making it promote our highest happiness to do right. But some one may say, "I am so wedded to my butter, and sugar, and pastry, and cakes, and they have so become second nature, that I cannot do without them." Well, if you cannot make the sacrifice of a radical reform, try a partial course, and you shall find a reward even in that. Take, for example, good, clear, light-colored wheat, and have it well ground, and kept in a close, tight cask, so that there shall be no need of sifting, and make from it unleavened bread, according to rule (Philosophy of Eating, page 46), or from good sweet yeast, and not eaten till it has been for some hours in pure air, to exchange its carbonic acid gas for oxygen, and use that, or rye and Indian, entirely, and a large majority will prefer it, at first, to fine white bread;

and though, at first, being harder of digestion, it may cause flatulence, yet, follow the rule for teaching the stomach to do its duty, and you will soon be rewarded in improved digestion and improved health. But in confirmed dyspepsia a more radical course will be needed; and in just the proportion as you return to natural food will be your enjoyment of digestion, your freedom from flatulence and colic pains, and you will find yourself able to do cheerfully all the duties of life. Hundreds have tried it, and this is their unanimous testimony; and if there are exceptions, they are only apparent, and are dependent on want of perseverance sufficient to overcome the effects of long-continued perversion of the digestive powers. At any time, before there is actual disorganization of some organs connected with digestion, which, from continued transgressions, will sometimes occur, a radical change, and conformity to Nature's laws, not only regarding food, but air, exercise, friction of the skin, &c., will effect a radical cure. (For other important considerations relating to digestion, see chapter on Leanness.)

THE DIFFICULTY OF OBTAINING NATURAL FOOD.

It may be thought impossible, in a fat and starch eating community like ours, to get a supply of natural food, and get it properly cooked. And in the deranged condition of the country, when half of all the grain raised is converted into whiskey and beer, and half of the other half deprived, by bolting, of many of its essential elements, and three fourths of all the milk is converted into butter, it might be difficult, at first, if we should all reform at once, to get a supply of natural food; but any man, or family, who sincerely desires to live according to philosophical principles, finds the means of doing so, and supply always follows demand in everything. But it is more difficult, especially in travelling, to get pure water, or the unfermented juices of fruits, to supply the liquids requisite to preserve perfect health; but this is not impossible, with access, as we generally have, to milk and fruits, which contain from eighty-five to ninety-five per cent. of water.

In Boston, where our water is almost as pure as distilled water, except where it is contaminated by contact with lead, zinc, or copper, in our service pipes and household appliances, and where we are blessed, the year round, with abundance of apples, pears, peaches, and other fruits, either fresh, canned, or desiccated, and all the meats, fish, vegetables, and grains that we ask for, and where we have, in most parts, clean streets, and well-ventilated houses, we might have almost perfect exemption, not only from dyspepsia, but from all other diseases, except, perhaps, those which come from external causes, as small-pox, measles, whooping-cough, &c. — and these would have no terrors for families who fortified their systems by the use of natural food and natural drinks.

The main difficulty is found in getting a constant supply of the unfermented juices of fruits, as, in the common mode of keeping them, they so readily ferment, when in contact with the air, that, though a cask or a bottle of purified cider or wine will remain unfermented while full, when a part is drawn out its place is filled with air, the oxygen of which produces fermentation. What we need is an arrangement by which the air shall be excluded from the cask or bottle as it is being emptied, and its place occupied by a medium containing no oxygen, or not liable so to impart it as to produce fermentation. Such a medium is carbonic acid gas, which is, luckily, of greater specific gravity than common air; so that being introduced into a room or vessel filled only with air, it will, like water, or any other liquid, rest on the bottom of the room or vessel, and exclude the air.

If these casks or bottles are placed in a small room or box, like a refrigerator, air tight except at the top, and that room or box is kept filled with carbonic acid gas, as we draw out the wine or cider the space will be occupied with the gas instead of air; and by the use of ice, these juices, and those of any other fruits or berries, may be kept the year round. On this principle, on a large scale, are constructed the fruit houses invented by Professor Nyce, in which are preserved the year round, apples, grapes, and vegetables, and by a slight modification, also meats, fish, and game of all kinds; while the more tender fruits and berries are preserved for a long time, so as to furnish a variety at every season of the year: and there is no difficulty of applying the principle, on a smaller scale, to any house or ship, at an expense not much if any greater than that of a common refrigerator of equal size. Indeed, in the greater convenience of taking out articles at the top, and saving the gas, the smaller preservator would have the advantage.

Does any one say he cannot afford such luxuries? Let any man calculate the expense of the butter and sugar and fine flour that is wasted in his family, and that causes, besides, the loss of his children, and the disease and suffering which these heating articles produce, — to say nothing of his expenses for sickness and doctors' fees, &c., — and he will find that he can have everything necessary to keep his family in health, raise all his children, fully developed in mind and body, have every luxury necessary to enjoy to the fullest extent all the gustatory pleasures of which he is capable, and have money left.

But what if there should be trouble and expense in

getting the necessary means of preserving health and furnishing all these blessings to his family, — could trouble and expense be devoted to a better purpose? There are certainly troubles and expenses in the evils and sufferings resulting from indulgence in unnatural luxuries, and from neglecting to furnish food and drink which are free from unhealthy qualities. In many places there is more trouble in obtaining water free from injurious elements than in obtaining food; and to save this trouble, men everywhere blind their eyes to the evils resulting from bad water, and make themselves believe that however others may suffer, their water is well enough; but all physicians know, and will testify, that any water, however clear and apparently pure, is unhealthy, and causes much disease and suffering, if it be hard, or contain any earthy, or mineral, or organic combinations. (See Philosophy of Eating, pages 190–205.) And yet almost all the world is drinking such water, and will drink it till it is absolutely undrinkable, rather than take the trouble to get good water.

In coral islands, where no drinkable water can be had, except rain from the clouds directly, and where it rains only a small part of the time, no expense is spared in catching and preserving that water, and I have seen arrangements for roofing and cementing cisterns for catching and preserving that water which cost the owner three times as much as the house he lived in.

It seems to be the design of Providence, that not only necessary food, but pure water, should be had only by the sweat of the face, and at great expense. And even the air we breathe is kept pure and healthful in cold climates by care and expense in ventilation, and in warm climates by care and expense in keeping streets and apartments cleansed from vegetable decomposition and all manner of impurities. And thus food, water, clothing, pure air, and all our blessings are furnished us only on condition that we work for them. But by a beautiful compensatory provision, our health and happiness are promoted by all these necessary labors; and they who are necessarily most constantly employed are most vigorous and healthy, mentally and physically, as well as most virtuous, useful, and happy.

Here we have the secret of the fact that the rugged and sterile soil of New England, Scotland, Switzerland, and other cold climates, have sent forth not only the muscles but the virtues and the brains which are needed to keep the world from stagnation and death. Everywhere the world over that people are most intelligent, virtuous, useful, and happy who are most constantly employed, and they most worthless and miserable who have most leisure time. And yet our national legislature have adopted the eight-hour system of labor, giving all the mechanics and laborers employed in every department of government work half their waking hours in which to serve the devil, who "always finds some wicked work for idle hands to do."

TASTE AND SMELL PROTECT THE SYSTEM.

We have seen that these senses, unperverted, direct us to wholesome food, and enable us to enjoy best that which is best for us, and, on the other hand, discover and defend us from that which is unwholesome or poisonous. For example: Good, well cooked fish, while it is fresh and wholesome, is invited and urged upon us by these senses; but let it remain but for a single hour in a hot sun, and they will inform us distinctly that it has become disorganized and unfit for digestion; and while unperverted they will thus always prove guardian angels to the system.

If poisonous, carburetted hydrogen gas escapes from our fixtures, even to the smallest extent, how soon do our olfactories detect it, and warn us of its danger! If a drain gets obstructed, and its contents flow back into our cellar walls, sending its death-dealing gases into our apartments, how kindly and quickly we are informed of the danger by the sense of smell!

If our cellars are damp and unventilated, and the fever and dysentery producing mould gathers on the walls and furniture, our olfactories never fail to warn us to ventilate and remove the cause of dampness, or we shall be sure to be sick and lose our children.

From such facts it is fair, and certainly safe, to infer

that every offensive smell is an angel of mercy, warning us to remove or avoid some evil influence connected with it, and inducing to cleanliness of person, and care of our premises, that we may avoid the evils that are sure to follow any neglect of such warnings. The importance of this subject warrants some further illustrations and facts, which go to show the importance of obeying the warning of the sense of smell, as in the cases above referred to.

The Importance of obeying the Warnings of the Sense of Smell.

From disregard to the testimony of this sense many a man has been made sick by eating fish, or other food that has become poisonous by the commencement of putrefaction and disorganization. And many a household have suffered in health, and have even been suffocated, by allowing gas to escape into their houses and sleeping-rooms. And the importance of neglecting obstructed drains and mouldy cellars is still greater, as is shown by the following facts: —

Some years since, a neglected drain, connected with a hotel in Washington, caused a terrible sickness, that prostrated for weeks some scores of the Congressmen and most valuable citizens, and; after a lingering sickness, the death of seven or eight, at least. And a similar cause, in a popular ladies' school in Pittsfield, induced severe and protracted sickness in many of the ladies, and the death of some, and for a time broke up the establishment.

Mould, however induced, — whether eaten in cheese, or mouldy bread, or other food, or breathed in the infinitesimal spora that are diffused from it in the atmosphere, — seems to be the source of a great variety of very serious diseases. One variety, which is found in the hold of damp and badly-ventilated ships, is proved to be the cause of ship fever, which is often very fatal.

Another variety, which is found in some localities, formed on newly-stirred earth, is the cause of fever and ague; and in one place at one time, in Western Pennsylvania, every man who worked in digging a canal was affected with it, and most of the inhabitants who lived in the vicinity, on low grounds, were also affected; but above a certain elevation all escaped; and on examination with a microscope, spora from mould on the recently-made banks, too fine to be seen by the naked eye, were found floating in the damp evening air in every house where those slept who were taken with the fever, but none in the houses on a higher level, where there were no cases of fever.

Other varieties of mould, in cellars and damp places, are believed to be the cause of typhoid fever, endemic dysentery, and many other diseases whose origin cannot otherwise be accounted for. These facts should make us afraid of all moulds, and, indeed, of all decomposed and decomposing materials, whether in the food we eat, or in our dwellings, or even in our vicinity, where they can impart to the air a deleterious influence.

As corroborating this view of the case, it is a significant fact, that in New Orleans, with more people in it than usual, for five summers, while the houses and streets were kept clean and clear from all decomposing substances, not a case of yellow fever occurred — an exemption never before known; and this, indeed, is almost proof positive that yellow fever is caused by mould, or at least by decomposition, with which mould is always associated.

SENSE OF TASTE A GUARDIAN ANGEL.

We have seen how the sense of smell not only invites us to what is good, but warns us against what is bad for us; and we shall find that the sense of taste was given for similar purposes. It not only directs us, as we have seen, to articles of food most wholesome at the time, and renders that most agreeable that is best for us, but it also gives us most disgust for that which would be most injurious. An animal, or a child, with unperverted tastes, may take in its mouth improper food, or a poisonous herb or drug, but it will be immediately rejected, and the more dangerous the article the more vehemently will it be disposed of. Give either of them a particle of tobacco, or alcohol, or opium, or any other drug, and you need not be in doubt whether these articles are intended for the benefit of the system.

This argument, together with the fact that I had never seen a disgusting drug, or an offensive article of food, do anything but harm, induced me, twenty-five years since, to resolve never again to allow a particle of food, drink, or medicine, that was offensive to the taste, to pass my lips. And I never have broken that resolution; and though I have had attacks of pain and sickness, as everybody else has had who has disobeyed the laws of his being, yet I firmly believe I have not suffered a pain more, or an hour of sickness longer, for keeping my resolution.

That, in health, our appetite and taste are intended to direct us to that which is good for us, and to protect us from that which is bad, in man as well as in brutes, is admitted by all intelligent physicians; and can it, at the same time, be true that, when sick and suffering, our heavenly Father, who, "as a father, pitieth his children," should intend to consign us to disgusting drugs for relief? That he should furnish us at all with means of relieving pains and sufferings induced by breaking his laws, is a miracle of mercy. But, beyond a question, it is true that the bitter and disgusting weeds and plants of the field each contain a principle adapted to the relief and cure of some suffering or disease. It is also true, beyond a doubt, that a law is given us by which, without dangerous experiments on the sick, we can ascertain what kind of pain or disease the remedial principle of each herb, or plant, or drug, is adapted to relieve.

By this test, the remedial virtues of some four hundred herbs, and plants, and drugs, — mineral, vegetable, and animal, — have been already developed and proved, more or less perfectly; and every one of them is found to do its work of mercy, if selected with judgment, with unerring certainty, and that in a preparation agreeable, or, at least, tasteless. And now I have come firmly to believe, that if any pain cannot be immediately relieved, and any disease cured, without offensive drugs, it is for want of knowledge of the right medicine, or of judgment to select and use it according to Nature's intentions. And this arrangement is in perfect accordance with Nature's general plan, giving us crude materials out of which, by the use of our intellects, to prepare medicines — just as we have crude materials out of which to prepare our food, clothing, &c.

Thus we see that all our wants, in health and sickness, are intended to be supplied without offending our natural tastes or appetites. The elements needed to promote the growth, health, or repair of the system, can be had in the grains, fruits, vegetables, meats, and medicines, all of which may be made agreeable to our tastes; and for sick children, or our feeble sons and chlorotic daughters, we need not resort to disgusting drugs, as iron, or phosphorus, or any other offensive medicine, to give health and strength, or to assist Nature in overcoming disease.

TASTE AND APPETITE PERVERTED.

WHILE it is true, as we have just explained, that an unperverted taste selects what is useful, and rejects what is bad, it is also true that a perverted taste often demands what is injurious, and rejects what is useful. We need, therefore, a test by which to try that sense. By comparing the analysis of the human system with analyses of different articles of food, as given in the Philosophy of Eating, we see that the grains, vegetables, and meats, in their natural state, all contain the same combination of elements and principles as are found in the system. And we have elsewhere seen that the unperverted taste of a child, or the taste of animals, directs, unerringly, to such articles as contain these elements and principles, in combinations best adapted to the wants of the system.

We have seen, also, that nothing is needed in the system but the elements and principles which are found in these articles of natural food, except pure water, and, perhaps, salt. That taste, therefore, must have been perverted which demands, or relishes, anything else than the principles thus organized; and, to prove it, we have but to offer any such articles as tobacco, alcohol, opium, or any crude medicine, to a child, or to any animal, and see with what disdain it is rejected;

but by mixing any of these articles, at first in small quantities, with something natural and agreeable, both children and brutes can be taught to relish them. It is worthy of remark, that, if left to themselves, no brute allows his taste to be perverted to a love for anything injurious; but if once induced to taste any such thing, will shun it ever afterwards.

I shall never forget the example of a hog belonging to my father, when I was a small boy. Some cherries, which had been soaked in rum, to extract their flavor, for making cherry-brandy, were thrown into his pen, and he imprudently ate enough to make him "gloriously drunk." Staggering about, and uttering silly grunts, he behaved as ridiculously, except in silly talk, as any besotted biped of the *genus homo*, and, finally, tumbled over, and went asleep. Being amused at his ridiculous behavior, I tried to induce him, afterwards, to reënact the farce; but not a cherry could he be induced again to take.

PREVENTION AND CURE OF CONSUMPTION.

WHEN we consider the delicate structure of the lungs, and the gossamer arrangement of air and blood vessels in which the air and the blood meet to perform their important vital functions, and that these complicated operations must go on, day and night, week after week, and year after year, for a lifetime, without stopping for rest or repairs, for a single moment; that the air and blood furnished them are often impure; that the chest is often so compressed that neither air nor blood are ever permitted to enter some of them, and that, consequently, they cannot have the exercise of their functions that is necessary to keep them in health; that parts of them are so often exposed to changes of temperature, by changes of dress, &c.; that their tissues are kept weak, for want of strengthening, nitrogenous food, and, at the same time, overworked, to dispose of extra heating, carbonaceous food, and, sometimes, excited by alcoholic and other stimulants; that when diseased they cannot stop to rest, and be cured; that means used for cure are more often injurious than beneficial, and that disease, when once engendered, is perpetuated, by transmission, from one generation to another, — when all these things are considered, the wonder is, not that eighteen or twenty deaths in every hundred, in all the civilized world, are of consumption, but rather that enough people live, anywhere, to perpetuate the race. Let us examine each of these sources of weakness, disease, and danger to the lungs, and get, if possible, some practical lessons from such examinations.

The delicate Structure of the Lungs, and the important Processes going on in them.

The air and the blood meet in a network of vessels, so fine that a powerful microscope can but imperfectly reveal its delicacy of structure; and in this wonderfully delicate network are constantly carried on operations so important that if, for a single moment, they stop, we faint, become unconscious and helpless, and, if they are not immediately restored, we die. In them oxygen is uniting with effete carbonaceous matter, removing it from the system, while using it for fuel to furnish animal heat, and, at the same time, imparting other important influences to the blood; and, whatever the condition of the lungs may be, these functions must be carried on without a moment's rest for repairs.

If the eye becomes inflamed, it is rested in a dark room till healed. If the muscles become inflamed, and rheumatic, and it gives us pain to move them, we lay them up for repairs, and keep them at rest till they can be moved without pain. But if inflammation attacks the lungs, and breathing becomes difficult and painful, however much we may desire to rest them, they must keep steadily on with their work, without a moment's rest, and, if healed at all, must be healed while hard at work. Another source of embarrassment, and cause of disease, is the bad material with which the lungs are compelled to work.

Impure Air and Impure Blood.

That carbonic acid gas is injurious to the system, and is a cause of consumption, we have abundant proof, and that, at every breath, the lungs give off this gas, in place of the oxygen consumed, is known and admitted by every one of common intelligence. It is estimated that, in a close room, without ventilation, a common-sized man consumes the oxygen, and replaces it with carbonic acid gas, at the rate of one gallon every minute, and, if he has access to no other air, will only live as many minutes as there are gallons of air in his room. Luckily, it is not possible to exclude all external air from our apartments, and, therefore, we are not absolutely suffocated while shut up in an unventilated room; but when we remember that every breath imparts some carbonic acid gas to the air, we can understand the importance of constantly changing the air in which we live.

And this importance is strongly enforced by the facts referred to in the Philosophy of Eating, page 336 — especially the experiment in the Foundling Hospital, and the Zoölogical Gardens, of London, where the length of life of infants and of monkeys were both doubled in two years, by a new system of ventilation; and, in this connection, it is particularly important to notice that the disease from which both infants and monkeys had died was consumption.

Here we have the explanation of the fact that consumption is more prevalent in cold climates than in warm. In warm climates, the houses being open, the air is being constantly changed and purified, while in cold weather, since fuel has become expensive, and open fireplaces have been discarded and close stoves substituted to save expenses of heat, the air is breathed over and over again; and even in houses of the rich, ventilation is disregarded, from sheer negligence. Many families also, especially among the poor, crowd together to save expense of heat, breathing constantly an atmosphere like that in which the infants and monkeys referred to died, before improving ventilation.

And many who feel it to be duty to have good air in the daytime, are afraid of the dampness of night air. But damp air is not generally bad for the lungs, unless it contains some malarious influence. Consumption is certainly no more prevalent in England where the air is moist, than in New England where it is comparatively dry. And, besides, we must either admit the night air to our houses and sleeping apartments, or breathe over and over again the day air that is shut up there; and it requires but a moment's reflection to determine which is best. Another source of weakness, and consequent disease of the lungs, is —

Compression of the Chest so as to exclude Air from some Parts of the Lungs.

The universal law, that every organ and every faculty must be exercised to acquire and retain its natural growth and vigor, as explained in Philosophy of Eating, page 337, pertains, of course, to the lungs; and the importance of the law is great in proportion to the importance of the organs to which it pertains. The lungs are contained in an air-tight chest, to which no air can be admitted except through the *trachea*, or windpipe. When the chest is expanded, as in raising the ribs for inspiration, the air, of course, rushes in to fill the vacuum, and passes through the *trachea*, and its ramifications, called bronchial tubes — which ramifications, growing smaller and smaller, till they enter and become a part of every point in the lungs, admit the air to every part, and give to every part a chance to assist in the performance of the duties of purifying the blood, furnishing heat, &c.

Now nothing can be clearer than the fact that if the ribs are tied down, or in any way prevented from being raised to the fullest extent possible, there must be some parts of the lungs into which the air cannot enter, and which must, therefore, remain without their natural exercise.

Very few, either boys or girls, are so dressed from their infancy as to allow access of air to every part of the lungs at all times; and our narrow-chested daughters, who entertain the ridiculous idea that a narrow chest and small waists are beautiful, exclude the air constantly from a considerable portion of the lungs, and the consequence is, as it must be, that the thin edges, from which the air is most perfectly excluded, are always the first parts to become diseased: so that when physicians examine the lungs and find these thin edges sound, they are quite sure all other parts are sound. Another cause of consumption is —

Eating too much Carbonaceous Food.

All the solid tissues, to acquire or maintain their health and strength, or to have recuperative power to resist and overcome disease, — as explained in Philosophy of Eating, page 16, and elsewhere, — must be supplied with nitrogenous food, in right proportions, constantly; but living as we do, and bringing up our children on too concentrated carbonaceous food, as I have before explained, all the solid tissues become weakened, and with them, of course, the membranous framework of the lungs; and this same carbonaceous food, furnishing as it does more work for the lungs in disposing of this extra carbon, overworks them, overheats them, and renders them more liable to inflammatory disease, and also, by diminishing their recuperative power, renders them less able to resist the encroachments of it; and these effects are increased by the use of alcohol, spices, and other stimulants. Thus the effects of excessive carbon in the lungs may be compared to excessive coal in a grate, which burns out the grate while it furnishes too much heat to the apartments; and this comparison is the more forcible in its practical application when we consider that, when burned out, the coal grate may be renewed, but the lungs, when once destroyed, are gone forever, and with them, of course, the whole system. Another cause of consumption is —

The Exposure of the Lungs to Changes of Temperature.

The point or apex of the lungs coming up, as it does, nearly to the top of the shoulder, is of course exposed to all the changes consequent on wearing low-necked dresses, exposing it almost directly to the cold, and then, perhaps, within a few moments, covering it with thick furs; thus at one time repelling the blood from the delicate structure by the contraction produced by the cold, and then suddenly inviting it by the expansion induced by heat.

At one time of course this part of the lung is shrivelled, so that very little blood is permitted to enter it, and at another, heated and expanded so that it is engorged with blood; and that these changes do have an effect, is shown by the fact that next to the thin edges, which are affected from causes before explained, these upper points of the lungs are always the first to become diseased in ladies, while in gentlemen, who usually keep these points covered, they are not more often found diseased than other parts. Another difficulty in curing the lungs, when diseased, is that —

The Means recommended for curing Diseased Lungs are more often Injurious than Beneficial.

The treatment of consumption, till recently, by the best physicians, has been merely a series of experiments; for a few months, by the recommendation of some celebrated medical man, or from the results of some apparent cure, using one set of remedies, and then, for a few months more, all going over to the plan of some other celebrity, and using something else, of perhaps entirely different nature. So, at least, it has been for the last forty years, since I have been carefully watching them.

At one time all the best physicians gave iron to strengthen the lungs and general system, and every chlorotic girl, and every boy with weak lungs, all over the country and the world, were taking disgusting iron pills — and that time has not yet fully passed away; and yet Trousseau, the highest authority perhaps in the world on this subject, said, some years ago, that "iron, in any form, hastens the development of tubercles;" and, "though it may induce a factitious return to health, and the physician may flatter himself that he has cured the patient," yet "to his surprise he will find the patient soon after fall into a phthisical state, from which there is no return."

At another time, Sir Francis Churchill recommends phosphorus, both to prevent and cure consumption, thinking that phosphorus is the element wanted for weak lungs — and all the doctors go into the use of phosphorus; but the doctor soon finds out, what he should have known before, that phosphorus is subject to the law that I have endeavored to explain, that all active elements are injurious, unless organized as food in some plant or animal; or, at least he finds that, unless great caution is used, some sad results are sure to follow the use of it; and now none who know the nature of phosphorus, but reckless doctors and bread-making chemists are not afraid to use it.

And the whiskey and cod-liver oil, which have been so extensively used, and still are so fearfully common, must be injurious, although they may sometimes induce fatness for a while, unless that philosophy shall prove to be false which I have endeavored to advocate, that it is not heat or stimulants that are wanted in weak or consumptive lungs, but nitrogenous elements, that shall give strength to the tissues and power to the system to overcome disease.

These opinions are corroborated by the fact now understood by every intelligent physician, that whenever consumption is cured, it is cured by the recuperative power of Nature, and therefore that cannot assist in any case which does not act in harmony with all of Nature's laws.

And now, considering all these predisposing and exciting causes of consumption, and adding the cause of general debility, induced by want of exercise in our ladies and sedentary men, and the fact that consumption, like every disease, may be transmitted from generation to generation, each becoming more degenerate as long as they live in disobedience to Nature's laws, can we wonder that eighteen or twenty deaths in the hundred in all the civilized world are from consumption? The wonder rather is, that enough live to perpetuate the race. And yet, if we carefully review these various sources of consumption, we shall find that every one of them is under our control and remediable, except, perhaps, the delicacy of the lungs and the necessity for their constant use, and even these, with the recuperative powers acquired by living according to the laws of our being, would not prevent their remaining sound during the time of our natural lives.

This is seen by the fact that other animals, with similar delicacy of organization, while permitted to obey their natural instincts, have not diseases of the lungs. Let us make such a review.

1. Is it necessary to breathe Impure Air?

With all the knowledge of light, heat, and the atmosphere which science now imparts to us, surely we can, if we will but take the trouble, make our houses light, warm, and comfortable, and have pure air to breathe every moment, night and day; and we can always avoid working in an unventilated room, or going into impure air, so as always to breathe air with plenty of oxygen, and without carbonic acid gas; and this could be had at an expense absolutely insignificant when compared with the evils which are induced by impure air.

2. Is it necessary to compress the Chest so as to exclude the Air from any Part of the Lungs?

I have seen a lady spend more than an hour, daily, in examining her house-plants, to see if no twig interfered with any other twig; that nothing superfluous remained, and nothing was wanted to develop the leaves, and branches, and flowers of any one. And she felt rewarded for her trouble if she saw them growing up healthy, symmetrical, and beautiful. With half that time devoted to her children, a mother could be sure that no form of dress, no string or belt, no habitual position in walking or standing, should interfere with the expansion of the chest to its fullest extent, so that at every breath the air would be admitted to every part of the lungs perfectly. And would not such a mother find a reward in the blooming health of her daughters?

I had hoped that increased attention to hygienic principles had overcome the absurd idea that a small waist is beautiful and desirable; and that mothers had come to consider what would promote the health of their daughters, rather than what would suit the fancy of addle-headed girls and their silly companions.

But I see, by a sensible notice in the London Spectator, that a book has recently been written in England devoted to the artificial production of the old spider waists of growing girls; — trying to induce mothers to mould their daughters by her standard, and never allow their waists to measure over sixteen inches; giving examples where fat, plump girls, with a waist of twenty-five or thirty inches, had been reduced to sixteen, and even fourteen; and giving a letter from one, in which she says, "All my torture is repaid by the admiration I excite;" and repeating over and over again that abominable falsehood and slander on men of common sense, "Men admire taper waists." The man that admires taper waists, with the feeble frame, and pallid and dingy face that always accompanies it, must be as silly as the brainless authoress of this ridiculous book. Think of a statue of Venus de Medicis reduced in the waist one third of its size from its standard twenty-five inches; or just for a moment consider the consequences that must follow from reducing the capacity of the lungs, aside from the consequences to the lungs themselves. The lungs, of course, are made of the right capacity, in proportion to the size of the body, to enable them to furnish all the oxygen that is needed to give life and vigor to the system, and no more; all the animal heat that is required to keep it in healthful glow, and no more; and to remove perfectly from the system the effete carbon, which, if not removed, makes the blood impure, causes the irregularities and sufferings so common, especially to the female system, and renders the complexion sallow and dingy, and the brain sluggish and inactive.

If the lungs are reduced one third, therefore one third of these life and health giving influences are lost; and, accordingly, in just the proportion as the lungs are reduced, we find cold feet, pains in the side and head, pallid and dingy complexion, with the fainting, palpitation, languor, and listlessness necessarily following — to say nothing of the weaknesses, pains, and irregularities of the abdominal organs, caused by pressure and displacement in compressing the ribs. And these are but a few of the natural and inevitable sufferings which come from this flagrant sin, aside from the more direct and fatal influences on the lungs themselves.

O, what can be sadder than to see mothers, in enlightened countries like England and America, where physiology is taught in our schools, thus sacrificing their daughters to the worse than heathenish god of fashion and false taste! For this class of mothers there is no hope; and the most merciful treatment of them is to consign them over to that beneficent law of Nature that makes it impossible, beyond a certain limit, for such consummate folly to perpetuate itself. Very few such devotees of passion live long enough, or have sufficient strength, to perpetuate their race.

But there is a class of erring mothers who are worth saving, and for whom there is hope — those who neglect their children from mere thoughtlessness; whose mothers allowed them to dress as they pleased, and who, in consequence, may have suffered a thousand ills and pains, but not having given the subject thought sufficient to trace these ills to their causes, and being still alive, think they do their duty to their children if they follow the footsteps of their mothers; but who, if once made to see their error, and its dangerous consequences, would be ready to do their duty, and thus save their children, and improve their race.

For the benefit of such mothers, I have pointed out some of the evils that might be avoided by allowing the lungs to be free, so as to be filled perfectly at every breath. And is it not reasonable to expect that young mothers of intelligence and education, or even of common sense, can be made to feel their responsibility in this matter, and be induced to set early about training their children, remembering that it is even more true in the nursery than in the garden, that "as the twig is bent the tree's inclined"?

The gardener who desires a symmetrical tree, sees that the little sapling is left free from the obstructions of weeds or shrubs, so that it can grow naturally; and if he neglects this precaution, he is sure to have a tree deformed and unsightly, as well as unfruitful and useless. And shall mothers allow ignorant nurses to put on the first dress of their little plastic infants with strings and bands, so compressing it that not the lungs only, but every internal organ is forced out of its natural position, and never, for a single day, allow those organs to assume their natural position? The ribs being turned inward, of course grow in that direction, compressing the lungs, and excluding the air from them; and a chest thus compressed at first will never expand naturally, even though corsets should never be applied to them.

Still, mothers who wake up to the importance of this matter, when too late to take the first step in the right direction, need not despair, if they will but do right afterwards, for Nature has wonderful powers to overcome difficulties, if she only have a fair chance. And they should be encouraged in this, as in other efforts at obedience. If they cannot, in their circumstances, obtain perfect exemption from all the evils described as consequent on compressing the chest and excluding the air, they will be rewarded by success proportionate to their efforts; and if, in addition to these efforts, they shall impress their children with the importance of this matter, the next generation will be greatly improved, both in beauty of form and vigor of constitution.

Why need the Lungs be exposed to Cold externally?

Here, again, you encounter the tyranny of fashion. And it is useless to preach to its devotees. What do they care for the fact that the point of the lungs exposed by low-necked dresses soon become diseased? Abiding by their motto, "as well out of the world as out of the fashion," they take each alternative; flitting, perhaps, like a butterfly, for a single season, in some fashionable watering-place, and then, having taken the other alternative of their motto, are missing. But, luckily for the world, they die too soon to be able to transmit their folly to another generation.

But there are those who are more devoted to the interests of their children than to the fashions and follies of life. Such need but to be shown the danger of any custom in order to abandon it. For such I am encouraged to write, with the hope that, showing them, as I have, the consequences of exposing any part of the body, and especially the delicate lungs, at one time to the open air, and at another covering them with thick woollens and furs, and that such habits cannot but diminish the chances of life, they will dress their children in accordance with laws of health, rather than with those of fashion.

How shall we avoid too Carbonaceous Food?

This, it must be confessed, is a difficult question. To resist the importunities of a kind-hearted old grandmother, with her pockets full of peppermints, is not an easy task for an affectionate daughter. She always gave them, as well as cakes, and pies, and good white bread and butter, to her children, and they did well. Ask her what is to be understood by doing well, and you will find, perhaps, that three out of six lived to grow up; and those who lived, not having had a fever more than once a year, or the colic more than once a week, and only such other diseases, and pains, and sufferings as it is *natural* for children to have, she thinks they really did well.

The grandchildren, therefore, are allowed a very little of cake or confectionery, with the determination, perhaps, never to permit enough to do them any harm; but, having once commenced, perverted appetite comes in to increase the difficulty, and the importunities of the child being added to those of grandmothers and friends, the young mother falls into the habits of others, trying all the time to make herself believe that it must be right and safe to do as every one else is doing. And if she ever wakes up to a sense of her terrible responsibility, it is only when some inflammatory disease has taken away her idol, or consumption has fixed on it its fatal seal.

But if mothers can be made to realize the truth, that children are liable to inflammatory diseases, and especially diseases of the lungs, in proportion as they use heating and stimulating food, of which butter, sugar, and fine flour are the principal articles in common use, and that they lose the recuperative power to overcome these diseases by the same means, these articles taking the place of the strength-giving nourishment of natural food, it seems to me they must break away from all such restraints of custom, and make it their first and highest duty to attend to the health of their children.

How can we know what Medicines to give and what to avoid?

If it be true, as I think I have proved it to be, that no one article of medicine is conceded to be useful in consumption by all, or even a majority of educated physicians; and if it be also true, as it certainly is, that all active medicines are conceded to be injurious if not useful, one important point can be easily settled by every intelligent man or woman, viz.: No active medicine should ever be taken with a view to cure consumption, for, according to the highest medical authority, it will be sure to do harm, while its chance of doing good is very small. And this is true, not only of the empirical nostrums so extensively advertised, but also of disagreeable drugs, however scientifically prepared.

That iron, which is so extensively used as a strengthening medicine, is not permanently useful, but very dangerous, is asserted on the authority of Trousseau, than whom there is no higher medical authority, who denounces the use of it as "criminal in the highest degree." That phosphorus, which was first introduced for the cure of consumption by Sir Francis Churchill, and which has been extensively prescribed in this country and Europe, is only temporarily useful, and permanently injurious, is asserted on the authority of two celebrated German chemists, Wochler and Frenich, who say that "phosphorous acid has a poisonous effect on the system analogous to arsenic."

That alcohol, which, in the form of whiskey, and in other forms, is now prescribed by hundreds of physicians, is not even temporarily useful, but, on the other hand, is permanently injurious, is asserted on the highest medical authority, including Dr. Bell of New York, who has devoted much time to the investigation of this subject; who is corroborated by Professor Carpenter of the London University, who says, "Alcoholic liquors do not mitigate the morbid effects of tubercle upon the system, in any stage of the disease, but, on the contrary, their use predisposes to tubercular deposition."

All the best physicians now agree that when consumption is cured, as it often is, even after it is confirmed, it is cured by the medical power of Nature. And those whom I esteem the best also agree that no medicines can assist Nature, except such as are prepared in an agreeable, or, at least, inoffensive form; but that in such a form medicines, judiciously selected, administered either in the usual way or by inhalation, do not only palliate uncomfortable symptoms, but often suspend the disease, even after ulceration has taken place, and the lungs heal up with a loss, perhaps, of part of their substance. Of such cases I have seen very many. By the exercise of reason, then, we can avoid medicines that will do us or our children harm, and can form some opinion of the class of medical advisers from whom to seek assistance.

If those who make medicine their life-study, and learn the nature of all medicines and all diseases, know so little, and so often do wrong, how dare we trust our lives and those of our precious children in the hands of quacks, who know nothing of the human system, nothing of the healing power of Nature, and nothing of medicine, except one, and nothing of that only that people have got well while using it, but do not know, as intelligent physicians know, that they got well in spite of, and not on account of, the medicines given?

Let us consider for a moment the chances of getting a medicine adapted to our particular condition at a given time, by taking it merely on the recommendation that it relieved somebody else supposed to be in the same condition. There are thousands of medicinal principles found in mineral, vegetable, and animal substances; indeed, everything not containing elements and combinations adapted for food, either for man or some other living creature, seems to contain a principle adapted to the relief of some pain, or to assist Nature in relieving some morbid condition of the human system.

No two medical principles have exactly the same effect, or are adapted to relieve precisely the same symptoms or conditions; and Nature has furnished us a test by which, without experimenting on the sick, we can judge what symptoms or conditions the medical principle of any crude substance is adapted to relieve. Let any number of healthy men or women — the more the better — take each an equal portion of any crude drug or vegetable, having any taste or active properties, and carefully note the effects, or symptoms, that follow in a given time, and they will be sure to find, on comparing notes, that at least three fourths of all who try the experiment will have some of the same symptoms or effects, varying according to age, sex, and temperament: and those of similar age, and sex, and temperament will have had a similar modification of symptoms.

Now let the least appreciable particle of the drug or vegetable thus tested be given to these or any other individuals of similar age, sex, and temperament, whenever pains or sickness, or other symptoms occur, similar to those produced by the drug or vegetable in the experiment described, and it will be sure to relieve such pains or symptoms. Experiments of this kind have been repeated thousands of times, and the principles involved are established as firmly as any philosophical principles ever were or ever can be established.

In this manner have been tested and recorded the symptoms produced by over four hundred different articles of medicine, and experiments are going on every day under the superintendence of some educated physician, in this and every civilized country in the world; and the field of investigation is so vast that these experiments may go on for centuries without fully bringing out all the medical resources of the world, and probably without finding any two medicines adapted to cure precisely the same set of symptoms.

Another fact has also been established by experiment, which at first astonished the doctors, but which, nevertheless, is proved to be true by experiments sufficient in number and accuracy to establish any truth, however unreasonable it might at first appear to be. This medical principle resides in every atom of matter of which any drug is composed, and exerts an influence in the cure of disease in the smallest particle in which the drug can be subdivided, as really if not as surely as in massive doses, but with this important difference: large doses of any active medicine may, if rightly selected, exert some remedial influence; but its good effects are more than counterbalanced by the harm produced on the principle already explained (see Philosophy of Eating, pages 160–167); while doses almost infinitely small, if rightly selected, produce the remedial influence without the evil.

Then consider how difficult it is to determine that a medicine is suitable for a given case, on account of the fact that it did good in some other case. How often, in case of cough, for example, we hear a certain article recommended because some other case of cough had been helped by it; but in nineteen cases out of twenty, on being tried, it fails, and for this reason: there are more than twenty articles of medicine that produce cough, as has been proved by experiment; but each one produces a cough differing in some respects from the cough produced by either of the other twenty different medicines, and each will cure its own peculiar cough, but no other. If, then, we take either of these twenty medicines at hazard, we shall have but one chance in twenty of getting a benefit from it.

Now suppose twenty persons are induced by an advertisement of a sure cure for cough, to try the medicine, and one of them is cured, while the nineteen are made worse, and some perhaps fatally injured by it. The nineteen will keep still, being ashamed of their folly; but the twentieth will tell all his friends and the advertiser, and get his name added to the list, to prove the remedy a sure cure.

But a skilful physician, who knew the characteristics of the cough which each of the twenty medicines is adapted to cure, would recommend at once the right medicine.

We see, then, how it is that more harm than good is done by medicines as usually administered, and how the good can be secured and the harm avoided.

Hereditary Consumption not necessarily fatal.

It is certainly a sad truth that "the iniquities of the fathers are visited upon the children to the third and fourth generation," but it is true, nevertheless, that the consequences of any transgressions of physical or vital laws do not stop with the transgressor; and yet there is great relief in the reflection, that except in congenital deformities, and organic diseases which are very rare, all that is inherited is a latent tendency to disease, which will never be developed if the child is brought up in strict obedience to Nature's laws, and that tendency will become weaker and weaker till it is eradicated from the system, or stronger and stronger till developed into fatal disease, as we obey or disobey the laws of life; so that, after all, each generation is responsible for its own diseases. There is evidence abundant that strong hereditary tendencies, and even the development of gout, apoplexy, and consumption, have been overcome and eradicated by strict adherence to the laws of life. (See chapter on Apoplexy.)

Let us now sum up the evidence in regard to the prevention and cure of consumption, and ask from the common sense of community a verdict on the question under discussion, — a question, I venture to say, which is more important, and interests more people, than any other question pertaining to this life.

Is it necessary that one fifth of our Race, or any considerable Part of that Number, should be sacrificed to Consumption?

The extremely delicate structure of the lungs, and the arduous and important functions which they ceaselessly perform, might seem to render it impossible that week after week, and year after year, such delicate and complicated machinery could be kept in repair; but we see that other animals, with lungs as delicate and functions as important, do have perfect lungs to the end of life, if, according to their own instincts, they are permitted to obey the laws of life; and it surely cannot be possible that man, the crowning glory of creative power, should have been provided with less perfect lungs, or less recuperative power, than the brute. Imperfectly constructed lungs cannot, therefore, necessarily cause consumption, and never do so if their natural recuperative power is preserved by obedience to the laws of life.

One, and perhaps the greatest predisposing cause of consumption, is breathing carbonic acid gas in unventilated apartments, as is clearly proved by facts to which I have already referred; but immersed, as every dwelling is, in a fountain of pure air forty miles deep, pressing on every side, and forcing itself into every crevice, and kept out of any room only by force, surely it is our fault if we do not have pure air night and day.

Another predisposing cause of consumption we have seen to be the exclusion of air from the thin edges of the lungs, by compressing the chest in the common mode of dressing infants, girls, and fashionable ladies, thus preventing the natural exercise of the parts involved, and causing them to become weak, and ready, like all other enfeebled organs, to take on a disease from the first cold, or other exciting cause. And is it asking too much of mothers, who value their children above all earthly treasures, to avoid this prolific source of consumption, by seeing to it that, from the day of their birth till they pass away from their responsibility, every part of the lungs of every child shall at all times be supplied with pure air?

Another predisposing cause of consumption is the alternate exposure to heat and cold of the upper points of the lungs, in consequence of dressing children and girls with low-necked dresses, and at one time exposing these delicate organs almost to the direct influence of the cold, and at another sweating them under thick furs; and surely no mother of common intellect can fail to see the unutterable folly of the excuse for which they thus sacrifice their children.

There is, however, a prolific predisposing cause of consumption more difficult to avoid, on account of the fixed habits of society — that is, weakness of the tissues of the lungs, and of the general system, induced by too much heating, carbonaceous food, and too little strengthening, nitrogenous, and phosphatic food, as has been explained in a preceding chapter, and also in Philosophy of Eating, pages 133–136. And yet I solemnly believe that any child whose mother has furnished it requisite elements for a perfect organization, and who has always had suitable elements for keeping the system in a healthy condition, without extra carbonaceous food, or other injurious elements or influences, will not only not be predisposed to consumption, but will have recuperative powers sufficient to overcome all other predisposing or exciting causes of this terrible disease.

If mothers could be made to realize the responsibility which this fact places upon them, they would, notwithstanding the embarrassments, overcome all difficulties, however great, and, breaking away from the starch and grease-eating customs of society, would say, with Joshua of old, "As for me and my house, we will serve the Lord"—by obeying his laws of life. And, as a reward for such service, they would enjoy pleasures in eating to which they had been strangers before, and also of seeing their children growing up in the beauty of perfect health.

But no one lives and sins not; and, in consequence of neglecting some of these plain laws of life, pains in the side, and cough, and inflammation of the lungs will occur. And it may not be easy, in such cases, to resist the importunities of friends to take some medicine advertised as sure cure for all pains and diseases, and, of course, adapted to *just such a case*, or which some friend had taken, and afterwards got better—most likely in spite of it. But if it be true, as

I firmly believe and think I have shown, that there are, at least, nineteen chances of doing harm to every one of doing good, surely they are safest who trust to the recuperative powers of Nature, with such harmless medicines as Nature provides, and gives us the means of testing, without these dangerous experiments on the sick.

Let any careful observer watch the progress of disease in the two classes of patients,—the one who resorts to every expedient recommended by every interested friend, trying to-day one kind of medicine, and to-morrow another entirely different in character and effects, going, in fitful mood, first to this doctor and then to that quack, without giving either time to do anything but harm, and the other class who use their reason and common sense in the treatment of themselves and their children, — and they will not fail to see these opinions corroborated.

Those who shift from expedient to expedient, taking everything recommended, and doing everything that anybody ever did in the incipient stages of consumption, are sure to go down, as Nature has no chance to exert her restorative power; while those who pursue a rational course, and adopt the simple, harmless, and efficient means which Nature has provided, if not neglected too long, are quite sure to recover, even now while the best of us know so very little of Nature's powers and resources.

I have patients in whose lungs have been tuberculous deposits for years, and some of whom were, when I first saw them, as really in consumption as their sisters or other members of their family had been but a few months before their death; and yet, by following suggestions like those before indicated, they have enjoyed comfortable health for years, and have not been obliged to deprive themselves of any substantial comforts or reasonable pleasures, except, perhaps, occasionally when cough, soreness of the lungs, and pain in breathing are induced by some exposure to cold, or other imprudence, and these attacks are soon and easily relieved by being properly attended to at once. And I have come firmly to believe that all cases of consumption, short of disorganization of the lungs, which render them incapable of performing the functions necessary to sustain life, and, indeed, all other diseases of which the human system is susceptible, are curable.

And the amount of disorganization that, by strict obedience to the laws of life, can be endured and overcome, is almost incredible. An intelligent young lady, the wife of a poor clergyman, came to me from the country, eight years ago, with one side of the chest collapsed, and one lung so far absorbed, or hardened, that not a particle of air could enter it, and the other main lobe inflamed and bestudded with tubercles in its edges and apex.

I had not the slightest expectation of her living but a few weeks; but, nevertheless, gave such directions and medicine as seemed to be indicated. In five or six weeks she returned, greatly relieved of her cough and inflammatory symptoms, but still panting like a frightened pigeon, breathing, at least, four times more rapidly than natural.

With the hopes of prolonging life for a while, and enjoying as much comfort as possible, she resolved to live on just such food and adopt such hygienic measures as I recommended. And I never saw her afterwards; but have recently learned that she is not only still living, but enjoys comfortable health; and, if careful not to overdo, or otherwise do wrong, is able to attend to all the duties of her station, and even, if occasion requires, to do her own house-work. And although she makes up in number what she lacks in the depth of her breathings, she is plump, and otherwise apparently healthy.

Such cases are exceedingly rare only because we rarely find patients willing to obey, strictly and perseveringly, the laws of life, or able to resist the importunities of friends, in such desperate cases, to take medicines that not only do no good, but seriously interfere with Nature's plan of cure; and rare, because of the utter ignorance, even among learned physicians, of the laws of hygiene. Not a medical school in the country, or any university with which it is connected, has a single professorship or course of lectures on that subject; and, humiliating as the confession is, I will not withhold the fact that I graduated at Harvard and practised physic for many years before I understood the first principles of it, especially of dietetics.

And, judging from the testimony of professors as late

as 1867, the advance in hygienic principles, in the forty years that have since transpired, has not been very great. At least, they have made no advances on Liebig's discovery, made thirty years ago, that "food is divisible into two classes — one respiratory, and the other nutritive." And, as Liebig had not learned that disorganized elements cannot be assimilated by the animal economy, so they continue to teach that disorganized and poisonous iron, phosphorus, and alcohol can be safely and advantageously used to give color and strength to the blood; to furnish a natural element wanting in fine flour bread, and to furnish respiratory food.

One of these professors testified, before a committee of the Legislature, that "alcoholic drinks act as respiratory food;" another, that "they have a proper use in the human economy, both dietetically and medicinally;" another, that the opinion of all the professors was in accordance with that already quoted.

One of these professors has obtained a patent for a process by which bread can be raised with phosphoric acid, and by which phosphorus can be imparted (as he says) to the system, in place of that removed in bolting flour. And all of them teach that iron can be imparted to the blood from the disorganized iron of the shops; and yet one author of their own text-books says "alcoholic liquids cannot supply anything which is essential to the due nutrition of the system," but that alcohol is "a stimulus, increasing, for a time, the vital activity of the body, but being followed by a corresponding depression of power, which is the more prolonged and severe in proportion as the previous excitement has been greater." And another author, perhaps more often quoted by them than any other, says of iron "that it hastens the development of tubercles," and denounces its use "as criminal in the highest degree."

In this advice and practice they also ignore the principle, now well established (see Philosophy of Eating, page 157), that disorganized elements cannot be assimilated by the human system. Of which principle, and of my position in regard to it, Dr. S. Dana Hayes, who finished his education in Europe twenty years later than these professors, says, "Modern investigations *certainly* sustain the ground taken that organized elements are the only ones assimilated in the human system."

Now, with teachings like these from the institution that claims to be the fountain-head of knowledge in this country, both literary and medical, is it strange that those who desire to find out, and are determined to pursue, the course that shall prevent or cure consumption, are utterly unable to be so sure that they are right as to be able steadily to pursue their course till their object is accomplished?

"Who shall decide when doctors disagree?" All intelligent men and women must decide for themselves and their children; and though it may, at first sight, seem exceedingly difficult, it certainly is not impossible for any one, who will give the subject the attention its importance demands, to decide correctly.

Not that every man must decide on all the details

of diet, regimen, and medicine that is needed, — that would be as absurd as to determine to make and mend his own watch, lest those whose business it is to do that work might do it wrong, — but decide as to the course to be pursued, not by the opinions of others, but by their reasons for such opinions; just as you found your hope of heaven on "the law and the testimony," and not on the opinion of other men, however learned or wise. But as in the one case you get instruction and advice from those who are themselves on the right road, so in the other you ask advice from those who have adopted the right course of treatment. Let us see if there are not

General Principles upon which we can come to right Conclusions in the Treatment of Consumption.

It is agreed, by all intelligent physicians, that medicines can never do good except as they assist Nature in removing diseases. Will Nature accept assistance from a crude drug or medicine which the natural senses of taste and smell, placed as sentinels to guard the system from dangerous intruders, loathe and reject? If not, crude medicines can certainly never be useful.

It is agreed that respiratory, or carbonaceous food, which includes oils, starch, and sugar, and, according to Liebig and the professors of Harvard College, alcohol also, furnishes no nutrition or strength to the system, but is useful only in furnishing heat and fat. Are cod-liver oil and whiskey appropriate articles for weak and diseased lungs? If not, how sad the mistake by which, within the last twenty years, thousands of hogsheads of these articles have been used, heating already inflamed lungs and adding to their labor, and especially in the use of whiskey, diminishing the power to perform it, thus hastening the process of decay!

Again, it is proved that phosphorus is necessary to give life and energy to the muscular and membraneous system, as well as to give action and energy to the brain, and that Nature has organized and distributed this element in the flesh of fish, active animals, the germ of grains, and mixed with nitrogenous food in greater or less proportions everywhere; and in order to prevent us from using this element in any other form, has made all disorganized phosphorus poisonous. (See Philosophy of Eating, pages 37–39.) Can we with impunity give crude phosphorus as a medicine, or use it in making bread, in place of the organized phosphorus lost in bolting wheat flour? If not, the seeds of consumption and other diseases are being sown broadcast in the community in phosphatic bread, patented by a learned professor, and recommended by him as perfectly harmless; and the doctors who have followed the learned French physician in the free use of crude phosphoric acid in diseases of the lungs, have made sad mistakes.

It is proved also that iron, organized and fitted for assimilation, is found in abundance in the food about us, both animal and vegetable; and to prevent our taking it in any other form, Nature has fixed a penalty for using disorganized iron. (See Philosophy of Eating, pages 160–163.) If so, Trousseau is probably right in supposing it to cause the development of tubercles, and in warning physicians against its use, as before stated. But are not our Harvard graduates doing a fearful business in recommending, as they do, everywhere, to all chlorotic girls, as well as to feeble young men, and, indeed, to everybody else who seems to need strength, some combination of crude disorganized iron, so that in almost all their families can be found a bottle of the vile stuff, and almost every day some member making up faces over it?

If to the foregoing considerations we add the fact, which I have endeavored to prove, that all crude medicines do harm, with but little chance of doing good, we shall have, I think, the means of knowing what to avoid as injurious in the treatment of consumption, or of predisposition to it.

Let us now consider the Course of Treatment from which we may hope to expect positive Benefit.

It is agreed that nutritive or nitrogenous food, which is found in some parts of all grains, the flesh of animals, and in greater or less proportions in all natural food, gives strength and vigor to muscles and all solid tissues, including of course the membraneous tissues or solid parts of the lungs; and it is agreed that weakness in any organ or tissue predisposes to disease of that organ or tissue. Nitrogenous food, then, and not that which is carbonaceous and stimulating, is the kind best adapted to prevent consumption; and inasmuch as this kind of food also increases the recuperative power of the system, it is that also which would best assist Nature in throwing off the disease when once commenced.

Again, it is found that animals which eat food containing most phosphorus are most active, and that birds of passage prepare themselves for their flight by living on seeds which contain most of that element (see Philosophy of Eating, pages 84–87), and that phosphatic food increases the action of the stomach and digestive organs, and indeed of all the organs and functions of the system. (See chapter on Dyspepsia.) Phosphatic food then, as well as nitrogenous, must be adapted to that dormant condition of the system, and the parts affected, which is always found with tubercular deposits, and all scrofulous diseases. Having, then, tables of analysis, showing the proportion of nitrates and phosphates in all articles of food in common use (see Philosophy of Eating, pages 121–126), we have the means of making selections adapted to different circumstances.

And then in regard to remedial agents, I have endeavored to show that Nature has provided in the weeds, and plants, and flowers, and in all the active combination of elements about us, mineral, vegetable, and animal, a remedial principle adapted to assist Nature in the relief and permanent cure of all the pains and diseases to which flesh is heir; so that our capacity to afford relief in all cases is only limited by our ignorance of the virtues of these innumerable agents, and our judgments in preparing and adapting them to the particular case under consideration.

And being provided with the means of testing the virtues of each remedial agent without dangerous experiments, and having tested, with more or less accuracy, some hundreds of these remedial agents, and recorded their virtues, we certainly have the means of assisting Nature with medicine, to some considerable extent, in removing the sufferings and overcoming the disease of even consumption, attended though it may be with more difficulties than any other disease which afflicts and destroys the human race.

And while the most careful students of Nature, and the wisest man, who, knowing the most of Nature's resources, and having most ability to choose and apply them, must be able to do the most that can be done in this terrible disease with medicines, yet, in view of all that is yet to be learned, he must feel, as Sir Isaac Newton felt in his last days of life — that all he had learned was but the gathering of a few pebbles from a single spot on some beach, while the borders of the boundless ocean were left unexplored. But after all, medicines are far less important than the recuperative power of Nature; and most of all who recover from consumption, recover in spite of medicines, and not on account of them, while many, if not the most of all who are lost, are lost because these restorative powers are prostrated or destroyed by the constant use of some deleterious medicines.

In conclusion, then, to sum up all in one sentence, we may enjoy perfect exemption from this terrible scourge, that consigns to the grave from one sixth to one fifth of us all, by breathing pure air night and day; avoiding compression, so that every part of the lungs shall always have its necessary air and exercise; avoiding too carbonaceous or stimulating food and drinks; careful protection from exposure to changes of temperature; and by keeping up the recuperative powers of the system by natural food and drink, appropriate exercise, and cleanliness of the skin. And if, by neglecting any of these precautions, consumption is threatened or ensues, if not neglected too long it may be warded off or cured by returning to neglected duties, and by using such medicines only as shall not interfere with, but assist the recuperative efforts of Nature.

INFLAMMATORY DISEASES.

How are they Caused, how Prevented, and how Cured?

WHAT constitutes an inflammation? The part first becomes irritated, and, according to a fixed law in the system, towards that irritation the blood flows, the natural secretions are increased, the minute vessels are distended or ruptured, and pain and soreness are the consequences of compressed or exposed nerves, whose minute ramifications extend to every fibre of muscle or membrane. These effects vary in different parts of the body, according to its structure, the pain being more or less severe according to the freedom with which the minute vessels can be distended; inflammations in the confined tissue of the finger, or confined parts of the hand, for example, are much more painful with the same amount of inflammation than unconfined muscles, which can be freely distended without pressing the nerves.

Active inflammations are known to be more prevalent in cold weather than in warm, and those parts are generally affected most which are most exposed to irritating causes. The mucous membranes of the throat, nose, or lungs are more often inflamed in winter, when exposed to the irritating effects of alternate cold and heat, — at one time to the air of a warm room, and at another time to the air at zero, — while in summer, and in warm climates, the digestive organs are more often irritated by the crude vegetables and fruits which are then more abundantly but not regularly used. But why do we suffer these inflammations, and the fever which accompanies them, while other animals, unless unnaturally restrained in their instincts and habits, are exempt from them? Let us see.

Nature furnishes three classes of principles in food for men and animals alike, — carbonaceous, which furnishes heat and fat; nitrogenous, which gives strength and health to the muscles and membraneous tissues; and phosphatic, which gives vital action to the nerves and brain. (See Philosophy of Eating, page 16.) These, in their natural state, are found in right proportions; and the instincts of animals direct them to food with these principles so proportioned as to be best adapted to their condition at all times and temperatures.

But man, whose instincts are intended to be controlled by his intellect, perverts his blessings by trying to make them better. He separates those principles from their natural. connections, in which they are prepared in exactly the right proportions, using those which he esteems the best, and rejecting the rest. In using fine flour, out of which is bolted the nitrogenous and phosphatic principles, he loses those which give him strength and activity, and takes only those which produce heat, and tend to produce inflammations.

In using butter also, which is the carbonaceous part of the milk separated from the other principles, he adds to his bread no elements of strength, but only increases its heating and inflammatory powers. Sugar, also, contains the same heating elements only. The fat of animals, and all vegetable oils, also contain no strength-giving principles, but are exclusively devoted to the production of fat and heat.

All these principles are necessary and healthful to the extent of four fifths of all our food; and if the food with which they are taken were deficient in these principles, they would not be unwholesome in their concentrated form to an extent sufficient to make up the deficiency. But our grains and meats, in their natural state, contain of these carbonaceous principles all that are needed; and all we add to them of butter, sugar, or starch is wasted, and tends also to produce unnatural heat, inflammation, and fever.

To make this statement perfectly comprehensible, even to those who know nothing of physiology, let us compare the process by which the carbon of fat, sugar, and starch are consumed to furnish heat to the system, with the process of combustion by which the carbon of coal and wood is consumed to furnish heat to our apartments, steam, &c. Indeed the processes are the same, except that the process by which heat is furnished by combustion from coal and wood is entirely a chemical process, while that by which animal heat is produced in breathing is a vital process, which cannot be explained.

As inflammable materials, therefore, are made more inflammable by constant exposure to extra heat, so the human system is made more susceptible to inflammations by exposure to extra heat from too carbonaceous food.

Many a steamboat has been lost because the sheathing and wood work around the boiler became so combustible, by constant heat, that the least spark ignited it — a spark that would have no effect on wood not thus heated and inflammable. So our lung fevers, catarrhs, sore throats, inflammatory rheumatisms, &c., are induced by exposures to colds and other slight causes, in those who live mostly on fine flour, butter, and sugar, while exposures to the same colds, and exciting causes of inflammations, have no effect on those who live on food containing only its natural proportions of heating principles.

And, to carry the illustration farther, as it is difficult to subdue the flames when once commenced on sheathing rendered excessively combustible by constant heating, so our lung fevers, sore throats, rheumatisms, and other inflammations, are obstinate, difficult of cure, and dangerous in exact proportion as the sheathing of the system is kept hot by carbonaceous food, alcoholic drinks, and stimulating condiments.

It is well known that the lower orders of the people of China, Burmah, and Hindostan, who live on rice, are afflicted greatly with low, inactive inflammations, especially of the eyes; and, by the table of analysis, Philosophy of Eating, page 123, it is seen that rice contains but six and a half per cent. of nitrogenous food to seventy-nine and a half per cent. of carbonaceous, while the standard article of grain — wheat — contains fifteen per cent. of the one, to seventy per cent. of the other. That this tendency to low inflammations is caused by extra carbon, is proved by facts which have come under our own observation.

Before the great rebellion in this country, which stopped for some years the supply of rice, the children of the Orphan Asylum, on Asylum Street, Boston, were fed, to a considerable extent, on rice and molasses; and they were greatly afflicted with ophthalmia, and at times nearly all the children had sore eyes at once. But after rice failed they were fed on oatmeal, hominy, and milk; and now, for seven years, have been entirely exempt from sore eyes, and have, in other respects, been manifestly more healthy and vigorous.

Observation also establishes the fact that gouty men are those who take little muscular exercise, and but little nitrogenous food, but living on fat meats and carbonaceous puddings, with rich gravies and sauces, and who also use, in some form, alcoholic drinks. Those, also, who are most subject to inflammatory rheumatism, and indeed to any inflammatory diseases, are those who live also on highly-stimulating, carbonaceous food and alcoholic drinks.

Here, then, we have indicated, not only the diet required to prevent inflammations, but also that which will assist in curing them; for if too much fuel has produced too much heat, it is clear that withdrawing the supply will help to cool off.

This Nature also indicates, in all grave cases of inflammations, by stopping the appetite, and making even the sight of carbonaceous food disgusting. She also indicates an important remedy, by giving us thirst for cold water. Thus Nature herself carries out the illustration of combustion, by ordering the fuel to be removed and the flames quenched with water.

In inflammations, then, and fevers, as in all other diseases and conditions, we can adopt no safer plan of cure than to follow Nature's suggestions. Withdraw all heating or carbonaceous food; then keep quiet, so that the blood will not be forced into the parts inflamed by active circulation, and especially that that organ or part inflamed may not be pained by exercise; then use freely cold water, as the thirst demands.

Then when nourishment is demanded, take such as is gratefully received, and never any other. These will always be found to be first the cooling sub-acid juices of fruits, like those of grapes, oranges, and luscious pears, or the soluble nitrogenous and phosphatic elements obtained from barley or oatmeal, or brown bread crust, which support the system without heating it; and these elements are best abstracted by soaking the barley or oatmeal in cold water, which, not coagulating the albumen, which is the principal strengthening element, allows it to flow out freely; but it should be boiled afterwards.

Then, as recovery progresses, the juices of the meats,

—those most agreeable to the taste always being best,—and, finally, in moderate quantities at first, return to the natural supply of carbonaceous and nitrogenous food.

In grave Cases of Inflammations and Fevers it is not safe to trust to appropriate Diet alone for Recovery.

Nature in such cases needs, and must have, to be sure of success, assistance also from the remedial principles which she has so profusely scattered around us, undoubtedly for this very purpose. This argument in favor of using medicines rationally, according to Nature's own intimations, as elsewhere explained, is, to my mind, irresistible.

The argument may be stated as follows: There are in the plants, and flowers, and active chemical combinations about us, medicinal principles which relieve pain, cool heated and inflamed surfaces and fevers, and assist Nature in the cure of diseases. This has been so often and so carefully tested and experienced that it is utterly foolish to deny it. It is conceded, also, by all intelligent students of Nature, that no elements or principles are created in vain, and that the uses of any element or principle can be determined only by knowing what it is capable of doing.

Having, then, these medicinal principles always at hand, and knowing that they are capable of affording relief, and having the means of knowing also what suffering each individual principle is capable of relieving, as I have explained, how can we resist the conclusion that there must be cases in which these remedial agents are needed?—else they are made in vain. And how can a consistent student of the laws of life refuse to use the means of relief so plainly revealed? And here, perhaps, as well as elsewhere, I may notice another error, likewise the result of a limited understanding of the laws of life, viz., that of adopting exclusively one class of articles of natural food, and rejecting others as always injurious.

IS ANIMAL FOOD ALWAYS INJURIOUS?

In the first place, it seems to me perfectly unreasonable that God, in blessing Noah after the flood for his faithfulness, should give him control of "every beast of the earth, and every fowl of the air, and all that moveth upon the earth, and the fishes of the sea;" and should tell him that "every moving thing that liveth shall be meat for you, even as the green herb;" and should cause to be deposited in all these living creatures the same elements, in the same combinations as are wanted in the human system, and as are found in the "green herb," or vegetable food, and should, at the same time, make one class to be appropriate food and the other injurious.

That each class of food does contain the same elements, in the same combinations, and nearly the same proportions, is seen by tables of analysis, Philosophy of Eating, pages 121–125. Take two articles — beef and wheat, for example. Beef contains of carbonaceous food thirty per cent., nitrogenous sixteen, phosphatic five, and water fifty. Wheat contains of carbonaceous food seventy per cent., nitrogenous fifteen, phosphatic two, and water fourteen. Now, considering that thirty per cent. of fat is equal to two and a half times as much starch, in heating power, or seventy-five to that of wheat at seventy, these two articles, the beef being of average fatness, in strengthening and heating qualities are nearly alike; but the beef has more than twice the nerve and brain food as the wheat.

In this last respect, however, beef and wheat differ less from each other than some other articles entirely vegetable. For example: Northern corn contains but one per cent. of nerve and brain food, while beans contain three and a half per cent., and Southern corn four. Where, then, is evidence, in chemical structure of animal, as compared with vegetable food, to show that the one is wholesome and the other injurious? And then as to the practical results of living exclusively on animal or vegetable food — where is found the proof of the advantages of the one over the other, either in the perfection and size of the body or in the vigor or length of life which they impart?

The Patagonian is the largest, and, perhaps, the most vigorous race of men, and they live almost exclusively on animal food, while the vegetable-eating Hindoo is a race among the most inferior. On the other hand, the vegetable, and milk and cheese-eating Bushmen are well formed, athletic, and vigorous, while the meat-eating Esquimaux are an inferior race of men.

And then statistics, while they prove, as I have shown in another chapter, that length of life, as well as health and happiness, depends on the free but temperate use of the good things that Nature has furnished, both of food and remedial agents, and on rejecting everything injurious in food, drink, medicine, or air, give not an item of proof that vegetarians live a day longer, or have less sickness or pain, than those who eat meat, but who live, in other respects, as temperately and carefully as their vegetarian friends. Nor has such proof been furnished from any other source.

That immense good has been done in hygienic and water-cure establishments, by taking patients away from their carbonaceous food, their stimulating drinks, and their death-dealing drugs, and giving them, instead, grains, vegetables, and fruits in their natural state, there can be no doubt. And that those who judiciously use, in addition to natural food, as some advertise, "pure air, water cure, Turkish baths, electric baths, electricity, galvanism, magnetism, gymnastics, movement cure, lifting cure, out-door exercise, social amusements," and even animal magnetism, whether under the name of mesmerism, clairvoyance, or spiritualism, are benefited in proportion as these remedial agents are judiciously applied, it is certainly reasonable to believe. And inasmuch as in such institutions there is less danger of doing harm by riding any one agent as a hobby, and using it for all cases, whether appropriate or not, as they are wont to do, who, knowing only one, believe in that only, that institution is safest and can do most good, other things being equal, which has at command the greatest number of remedial agents.

My ideal establishment, and one to which, when other things fail, I should like to go, or send my friends, is one in which are at command all the resources of Nature, both hygienic and remedial, including, of course, "living things that move" as well as vegetables for food, and the medical principles which are provided in the weeds, and plants, and flowers in the fields about us; and in which also are to be found men of good common sense, who understand the nature of all these varieties of food and medical principles, and their adaptation to each particular case that comes before them. Every one of these alimentary and remedial agents is sometimes needed, else it would not have been provided; and he who uses water cure alone, or electricity, or any other one of all these remedial agents, must be as narrow minded as he who believes that man should "live on bread alone," and that all other food was made in vain.

It is lamentable, and yet amusing, to see how minds are narrowed down by confinement to a little circle of thought, as in the study of one or only a few of Nature's resources. In 1832, when all minds were exercised with thoughts on Asiatic cholera, I had two patients whom I visited daily for some time. One was a chemist, who made nitre and sulphuric acid, and, of course, studied oxygen, and the other an organ-maker, who studied air. As they became convalescent, so as not to think exclusively of themselves, they amused me daily each with his own "theory and practice" in cases of cholera, and indeed in most other diseases.

The *chemist* thought that want of oxygen in the air must be the cause of cholera; and he made the proof of the theory clear, to his own mind at least, by considering the facts that oxygen was the element which gave purity to the blood, and life and energy to the system, and that cholera was a disease of depression, and cholera patients turned blue, also, just as drowning men do, for want of oxygen.

The *organ-maker* thought cholera must be caused by confined air, for men who were suffocated in confined air had very much the appearance of those suffering and dying with cholera; and he had no doubt that if cholera patients could be carried directly into the wind, they would soon recover.

The *water-cure doctor* makes himself believe that water, cold and hot, in its varied applications, is the only remedial agent needed in the cure of any disease.

The *electrician* thinks electricity the source of life; and all that is wanted in any disease is to regulate and control electrical currents, and therefore water must be carefully avoided, lest it should interfere with the cure, for even damp air is death on electricity.

The "*lifting-cure*" *doctor*, who knows nothing else, seems to believe that not only muscular power, but recuperative power, and even brain power, are proportionate to the number of pounds he is able to lift. And though one third of his power may be gained by yoking himself like an ox, yet if in that way he can lift three thousand pounds, while without a yoke the strongest man never raised but a ton, he seems to fancy himself one third stronger, healthier, and wiser than the strongest man who never dignified himself with the yoke.

And even some of those who style themselves *rational practitioners* seem not to have much broader views of the medical resources of Nature; for while there are hundreds of medicines which can, and, if rightly administered, do, assist Nature in the relief of pains and the cure of disease, and which must, therefore, have been given us for that purpose, the professor of *materia medica* in Harvard College tells his class, every year, "If I can have *four*, or at most *six*, medicines, I can cure all diseases and relieve all pains that medicines are capable of curing or relieving."

My definition of a rational practitioner is he who, despising or rejecting none of the provisions of Nature, hygienic or curative, as far as possible follows the sacred injunction, "Prove all things; hold fast that which is good."

CONSUMPTION OF THE BLOOD.

THAT peculiar greenish or ash-colored appearance which is seen in our feeble, undeveloped daughters, and which indicates the disease called chlorosis, from the color of the skin, — being a watery state of the blood, — is supposed to be caused by want of iron in the system; and hence such girls are always found taking iron, in pills, or drops, or in some other crude preparation, with the vain hope of thus restoring iron to the blood. And as, for a while, the appetite is improved, and the strength apparently increased, the remedy is continued; but the improvement is deceptive, and never, according to my experience and observation, effects a permanent cure. And this opinion is confirmed by the highest medical authority, as I have quoted before. (See Philosophy of Eating, page 161.)

One sentence from Trousseau is so important in this connection, that I will repeat it here, there being no higher authority on this or any other medical subject. As quoted by J. Francis Churchill, a celebrated French physician, who confirms the statement, "M. Trousseau declares that iron, in any form, given in chlorotic affections, to patients in whom consumptive diathesis exists, invariably fixes the diathesis, and *hastens the development of tubercles*. The iron may induce a factitious return to health; the physician may flatter himself that he has corrected the chlorotic condition of his patient; but, to his surprise, he will find the patient soon after fall into a phthisical state, from which *there is no return*. This result, or at least its hastening, M. Trousseau attributes to the iron. The assertion is a most startling one. M. Trousseau is nevertheless so certain of what he says, that he denounces the administration of iron in chlorosis as *criminal in the highest degree*."

No attempt has ever been made, to my knowledge, to refute the opinions of these two celebrated physicians, and it corroborates the doctrine that I have elsewhere endeavored to establish (see Philosophy of Eating, page 159), that "no elements are allowed to be incorporated into and become a part of the blood, in any organ or tissue, that are not fitted for digestion in some vegetable," but that, on the other hand, they become poisonous or injurious to the system. And yet, if you ask the first ten green or ash-colored girls you shall meet, what they are taking as medicine, nine will probably tell you iron.

And the most of them, if they have taken it but a short time, will declare they feel better for it. And this is accounted for on the same principle that alcohol, another article composed of disorganized elements, deceives the feeble patients who take it, by making them at first feel better, but afterwards, as the stimulus loses its power, depressing them in the same proportion as they had been stimulated. Iron, however, is a slower and more permanent stimulant, and therefore more deceptive. For a time, however, like alcohol, it increases the powers of digestion, and causes, perhaps, iron to be appropriated from the food; for sometimes the color of the cheeks and the blood return, and it apparently becomes thicker and better; but that the strength and color of the blood in that case are produced by the stimulant, and not from the iron directly, is proved by the fact that alcohol, and phosphorus, and some other stimulants, will do the same thing, and even quicker than iron. In all cases, however, these stimulants leave the system more depressed at last, and thus hasten the development of incurable consumption, either of the lungs or bowels.

What is the Cause of Chlorosis?

I have investigated scores of cases, and found their history to be uniformly the same. From the time of its birth, and months before, till the child was weaned, the mother had lived on food which contained very little iron, or any of the elements of which its tissues or blood is composed.

Butter contains not a particle of iron, sugar none, and superfine flour very little. (See Philosophy of Eating, pages 29, 30.) And yet I have found many a young mother whose principal food consisted mostly of white bread and butter, cakes, pastry, confectionery, and coffee and tea, neither of which, nor all together, would contain, in all she could eat, of iron, phosphorus, nitrogen, or lime, sufficient to make blood, bones, or muscles in good condition for the child alone, while her own system would be left unsupplied.

It is a curious physiological fact, that in such cases Nature provides first for the child, and if the expectant mother fails to supply elements sufficient for both herself and the child, the child will be first supplied at the expense of the mother; and we often see white bread and butter, and cake and pastry-eating mothers pale and feeble, and suffering intensely from defective teeth and neuralgia, for want of iron, phosphorus, nitrogen, and lime, while the infant may be born in a condition comparatively well developed and healthy.

And then in nursing, though the child gets the best of the elements furnished, still it can never get good blood from such food as does not contain the elements of good blood; and when it is weaned, its food will probably be of the same kind as that on which its mother lives. And thus if it lives at all, it will grow up feeble in muscle, for want of nitrogen; defective in teeth, for want of lime; neuralgic, nervous, and hysterical, or perhaps stupid, for want of phosphorus; and pale and ash-colored, for want of iron. Such are the girls who have a morbid, indefinite craving for something, they know not what, and therefore add to their troubles by eating such unnatural and abominable things as chalk, slate pencils, magnesia, pickled limes, &c., their systems being deficient in important health-giving elements.

I once made a post-mortem examination in case of a chlorotic young lady, who died after intense and long-continued sufferings, the cause of which could not be ascertained while living; and we found a ball of magnesia that weighed a pound, and other smaller ones, embedded in the intestines, obstructing the passage, and finally stopping it altogether. And there are numerous records of similar cases. And if they do not thus accumulate, all unnatural or undigested articles in passing off must produce irritation, and tend to develop tubercles of the bowels and other diseases. Having, then, the cause of this disease, or at least the foundation of what is called consumption of the blood or bowels, as well as consumption of the lungs, to which so many of our daughters are sacrificed, it is certainly an important inquiry, What will cure this terrible malady?

What is the rational Mode of curing Chlorosis?

If my position is true, that chlorosis is simply the want of iron and other necessary elements in the blood, and if it be also true, as I have elsewhere endeavored to prove (see Philosophy of Eating, pages 9–13), that these elements are all furnished and at hand in "every herb bearing seed, which is upon the face of all the earth, and every tree in the which is the fruit of a tree yielding seed," and also in the flesh of "every beast of the earth, and every fowl of the air, and everything that creepeth upon the earth wherein there is life," which, having obtained in their flesh the elements as organized in the herb, and the seed, &c., and being thus fitted to be food for man, were given to Noah and his posterity as a blessing, for food, "even as the green herb;" and if it be also true, as I think I have shown, that neither iron, nor any other element not thus organized, can be assimilated as an element of the blood, but, on the other hand, is interdicted as poisonous, — then surely the rational mode of cure is clearly pointed out. We have but to take food freely which is known to contain iron and other elements as they are needed.

But how can we ascertain whether any Elements are wanted to make the Blood pure in any given Case, or, if so, what are the deficient Elements of the Blood?

Why not use common sense, as our mechanics and chemists use it in their every-day operations? Suppose an intelligent soap-maker should find that a lot of soap, which a blundering man had attempted to make, was good for nothing because the necessary elements were not mixed in the right proportions, — how would he ascertain what was wanted to make good soap of it? Knowing just how much alkali and how much oil or grease were necessary for the quantity before him, he would ascertain how much of each had been used; and if a pound of potash was wanting, would add it to the mixture; and if other necessary conditions were complied with, he would be sure of good soap. But suppose he should not know what was needed, and should add at hazard a pound of grease instead, would he get good soap?

Upon the same principle, if we see a feeble, sickly,

undeveloped girl, without disease of any particular organ, we know that something must be wanting in the blood; and what that something is, we can know by ascertaining what she has omitted to supply. If she has lived principally on superfine flour bread and butter, or cakes and confectionery, or any other food of which starch, butter, or sugar is the predominant principle, we know that she has omitted to supply her blood with iron, nitrogen, phosphorus, lime, &c., as these articles of food do not contain these elements. What, then, does common sense dictate, in such a case, but to omit such articles of food, and take instead such food as is known to contain these deficient elements? Just as, in the supposed soap case, the intelligent soap-maker omitted the grease and added alkali.

A woman in the country once gave me an account of what she called her bad luck in attempting to make soft soap. She put together, as she thought according to rule, her grease and lye, and boiled them, and added the right quantity of water, and stirred it; but the soap "wouldn't come;" and not knowing what was the trouble, she asked a neighbor, who told her she had heard that salt was good, and advised her to add a pint of salt, and stir it all day. She followed the advice, and still it wouldn't come.

She consulted another neighbor, who told her the trouble was, that she stirred it a part of the time one way and a part of the time the other, and thus undid at one time what she did at another: she must stir it always with the sun, and that would certainly fetch it.

"She stirred it, and stirred it; but the more she stirred it the more it wouldn't come." Finally she consulted a very old and experienced housekeeper, who assured her it would come if she stirred it when the sign was right. She must get old Isaiah Thomas's Almanac, and look up the signs of the zodiac, and when the sign was right she must stir as before directed, vigorously, with the sun, and her trouble would soon be over. She followed advice, but after all lost her soap.

Now, absurd and ridiculous as were these whims of the grandmothers of the past generation in regard to the making of soap, they were not a whit more absurd or ridiculous than those of the mothers of the present in regard to the treatment of what are called humors, or impurities of the blood, especially of that condition of which we are now treating, and from which so many of our daughters are lost. Indeed, that mother is a rare exception who, after iron has failed, does not resort to beer, or wine, or oxygenated bitters, or some medical discoveries, or something else which some neighbor or quack doctor shall tell her is good for the blood, although not one of them all has more power to cure chlorosis, or to purify the blood, than the signs of the zodiac have power to make soap; but they have more power to do harm, and that harm is incalculably more important. And yet, to carry out the illustration, it is no more certain that good soap can be made without failure by using the right materials in the right way, than it is certain that pure blood can be made by the right use of the elements which constitute good blood.

But what kinds of food contain iron? Analyses of different articles have not yet been made to determine the proportion of iron which each article contains; but a general statement will be sufficient for all practical purposes. The flesh of all animals contains iron, and of course milk, grains, fruits, and vegetables, which make the muscle or flesh of animals, contain it.

Iron, phosphorus, lime, and all other mineral elements, are connected together with nitrogen, for making muscles and blood, but not one is found connected with carbon, which furnishes fat and heat, so that those articles of food which are found in the tables to contain the most nitrogenous and phosphatic elements generally contain most iron. (See Philosophy of Eating, pages 121–125.)

To prevent chlorosis, therefore, mothers have only to see that their daughters always live on food containing all its natural elements; and to cure it, they have but to select the articles of natural food which contain most phosphatic elements.

VIGILANCE IS THE PRICE OF HEALTH.

SEEING among the barefooted and neglected children in the streets more vigor and health than among the better classes of children, we might at first sight conclude that children most neglected were most healthy; but looking into the matter, and learning facts, we find that the robust only are seen in the streets, because all the rest are dead and buried, and out of sight: while children among the better classes are kept alive in spite of puny frames, flabby muscles, pale faces, and miserable carbonaceous diet, by better care in regard to air, warmth, cleanliness, &c., in their houses, and especially in their sleeping-rooms, as well as by less unwholesome food.

Look at the bills of mortality in Boston, week after week, the year round, and you see that more than two of foreign birth die to every one of American; and yet the foreign population are not as numerous as the American. And this is not a full illustration of the importance of obeying Nature's laws, for many American citizens live in the same degraded and neglected condition; but their deaths being recorded with those of American born, diminish the contrast.

And on the other hand, many foreigners live as carefully as Americans; and their deaths being recorded with those of foreign-born citizens, diminish also the contrast. What can account for this fearful mortality among the neglected poor but disobedience to Nature's laws?

In winter they breathe the air over and over again, because they cannot afford fuel necessary to give ventilation, and are also poorly protected from the cold. And in summer they breathe air also contaminated with impurities from neglected drains and vegetable and animal decomposition, because in such localities rents are cheap. And then, for the same reason also, they live on stale vegetables and fruits, and other unwholesome food.

Of course, under these circumstances they are much more liable to be sick, and when sick, are almost sure to die; and the wonder to me is, not that so many die, but that any should be tough enough to live. But this class of population is terribly prolific, as well as terribly mortal, and on that account fears have been expressed lest they should outnumber and control the better classes. But a little attention to facts will dissipate all such fears.

My attention was first called to this subject thirty-five years ago, by some statistics gathered by a Swiss gentleman, named Francis D'Ivernois. This gentleman was preparing a book on European statistics, &c., when a writer named Morrow D'Jannes, discovering the fact that in a miserable, semi-savage Russian province the number of births far exceeded in proportion those of other European nations, and making the same mistake as that to which I have referred, wrote an alarming pamphlet to prove that the time would come when these miserable Russians would overrun all Europe, and control its destinies.

D'Ivernois, seeing the blunder of D'Jannes, published what statistics he had collected on this subject, and proved to my mind that a degraded and neglected people, however prolific, can never outnumber or overcome a virtuous people, who take care of themselves. There may be found among them the hardy and robust, because such are too tough to be killed by any neglect or abuse, as is seen in the low classes in Boston to which I have referred, and among our native Indians, who seem hardy and robust, while their race is dying out. Still a merciful Providence has kindly provided that beyond a limited extent misery cannot perpetuate itself; while they who live virtuous lives, and best take care of themselves, have the best average amount of health and the greatest average length of life.

D'Ivernois first compared the people of this miserable Russian province with the Swiss people in the canton of Vaud. The Russians were miserably fed, badly housed, and badly provided for in everything that pertained to the comforts of life; while the Swiss parish, under the care of a worthy dean, were comfortable, virtuous, contented and happy, living on a generous diet of such meats and vegetables as by industry the country was made to produce.

The births in Montroux, the Swiss parish, were one to forty-five inhabitants, while in the Russian province they were one to seventeen. But in Montroux only one died in every sixty-four, while in Russia one died in every twenty-five. So that, notwithstanding the frightful number of births in the Russian province, the Swiss gained in population the fastest.

But supposing it possible that this result might be dependent on the difference in climate, he compares the same Russian statistics with those of Leysin, a parish among the Alps, where the people lived on the natural food of that rugged region, obtained by industry and hard work, and were also a virtuous, contented, and happy people. Here the proportion of deaths was somewhat greater than in the remarkably healthy parish of Montroux, but still they were less than half as numerous as among the Russians, although their climate was vastly superior to that of the Swiss. And these are but samples of facts which go to establish my position.

At the time these statistics were gathered by D'Ivernois, I collected what I could to show the chances of life in America as compared with those in Europe and other countries; and from old rusty minutes of a lyceum lecture, written in 1833, I make the following extracts: —

"In our own country, especially in our own happy New England, very few ever suffer for want of food; and probably no people in the world are more virtuous, or take better care of themselves. From the landing of our Pilgrim fathers we have eaten liberally of meats, grains, vegetables, and fruits, in their natural state, and if we look the world over we shall find no people a greater proportion of whom have lived to old age, and no people have increased more rapidly in a healthy population. It is much to be regretted that our statistics are so imperfect; but imperfect as they are, we may yet derive from them decided evidence of the wholesome qualities of good beef and pork, with Indian corn, rye, beans, with other vegetables and fruits, cooked with Puritanic plainness, and eaten with the relish which a virtuous and industrious life always give to natural food.

"In Montroux, the most healthy parish in Europe from which statistics have been taken, one died in sixty-four, as before stated. In all the New England States the deaths only average one in seventy-five; so that our prospect of living to the age of sixty is twenty per cent. better than the people of the most healthy parish in Europe. And surely our climate is not better than that of Europe, especially that of Montroux, which is situated in a remarkably pleasant valley at the foot of the Alps. Let us look also at the people of other countries, and compare our statistics with theirs.

"In Batavia, the deaths are one in twenty-six; in Trinidad, one in twenty-seven; in Martinique, one in twenty-eight; in Bombay, one in twenty; in Havana, one in thirty-three. So that we find that the deaths in these countries are on an average nearly three times more numerous than in New England. We find by these statistics, that in the countries where the people are the most miserably fed and cared for, the average length of life is shortest; while those which approximate most nearly in regular, virtuous habits, and in the comforts of life, to New England, approximate to us also in the average length of life."

Whether or not our statistics will compare now with other countries as favorably as they did thirty-five years ago, when the above was written, the deductions from the facts are valuable, establishing, as they do, the doctrine that that people live the longest, and enjoy the best health, who take best care of themselves, and live most nearly in accordance with Nature's laws.

HOW TO PREVENT APOPLEXY, NEURALGIA, AND NERVOUS DISEASES.

If you look at the analysis of the brain and nerves, Philosophy of Eating, page 87, you will find them composed of albumen, a fatty substance called cerebral fat, phosphorus, mineral salts and water; and that the mature, healthy, adult brain contains more albumen, more phosphorus, and more mineral salts, but less cerebral fat, and less water than the brain of infants or idiots.

The elements that are thus shown to be needed are found in all natural food, combined with nitrogenous, or muscle-making principles, but not with the carbonaceous, or heating principles; in milk, and eggs, and fish, and the grains, &c., in their natural state, but not in starch, any fatty substance, or sugar. Those, therefore, who live mostly on white bread, butter, and confectionery, which contain none, or very little of these elements which keep the brain and nerves in a healthy condition, are those who suffer most from headaches, neuralgia, and nervous diseases, and those who, finally, die of apoplexy.

We have noticed, also, in another chapter, that nursing and expectant mothers, who live on carbonaceous food, are peculiarly liable to toothache, headache, neuralgia, and nervous disorders, because Nature favors the infant at the expense of the mother, and therefore, if the right elements are not furnished sufficient for child and mother, the mother suffers first. These hints clearly indicate the course of diet necessary to prevent headache, neuralgia, nervous excitements, apoplexy, and all other diseases dependent on the healthy action of the nerves or brain; and this on the simple principle, so often explained, that no organ or function can perform its appropriate duties, or keep in health, without a constant and regular supply of the elements composing or used in that organ or function.

For all these sufferings from headache, neuralgia, hysterics, &c., from which the young suffer so much, and many so intensely, the remedy is simple and certain. Avoid the heating, unnatural articles of food, out of which have been taken the elements before enumerated as necessary to keep the brain and nerves in order, — such as white bread, butter, fat, and sugar, and all the pastry and confectionery which are made up of those heating principles, — and take, instead, only natural food, in which are retained the elements needed, and the cure is certain.

Apoplexy, also, which seldom, I think never, occurs except in those who have been for a long time overfed with carbonaceous food, almost never occurring in persons under forty years of age, and not in persons so young as that, unless they have added to carbonaceous food the stimulus of alcoholic drinks or strong spices and condiments, is, of course, prevented by abstaining from the articles which cause it, and taking, instead, those which contain the elements necessary for the healthy action of the brain.

My attention was, many years ago, particularly directed to this subject from motives of strong personal interest in it; and I have often had occasion to prescribe for others the course that I have found useful to myself, with a success which fully confirms me in the view of the subject just given.

At the age of forty my father commenced having premonitory symptoms of apoplexy, and from the age of forty to fifty had a number of slight attacks, and one quite severe; but he made no change in his habits, eating habitually highly-carbonaceous food, and drinking, as the custom then was, brandy, or some other alcoholic drink, three or four times a day, and, at the age of fifty-four, he died suddenly of apoplexy. At the age of forty I also, having inherited his form and constitutional characteristics, commenced having the same kind of premonitory symptoms of apoplexy, which also continued and increased till after the age of fifty, although, supposing then that that was all that would be necessary, I abstained from all alcoholic drinks and stimulating condiments; but having an attack that rendered me unconscious for an hour or more, I found something more was necessary to save me from my father's fate. After that I gradually diminished my carbonaceous food till I came up, I think, to the true philosophy of eating; and now, at the age of sixty-four, I have, I think, eradicated all hereditary tendency to apoplexy, not having had, for some years, even a headache, or other premonitory symptom of it; and, besides having disposed of other infirmities, I have more energy, more power of endurance, mentally and physically, and more recuperative power, than I had at the age of forty.

My son, also, at the age of thirty-six began to have the same premonitory symptoms as his father and grandfather had before him; but, by abstaining from stimulants and carbonaceous food, has in two years quite overcome them. And I make the sacrifice of publishing these personal items in hope of benefiting others who may have similar hereditary tendencies, and in the hope of corroborating, if not confirming, the opinion elsewhere expressed, that hereditary diseases are not necessarily incurable, or hereditary tendencies eradicable.

THE CAUSE AND PREVENTION OF DEFECTIVE TEETH.

In one important respect the teeth differ from other organs of the animal economy — they have no recuperative power. But, to compensate for this defect, they are made of materials more indestructible than those of any other organs; so that being properly supplied with the elements requisite for their formation and nourishment, and used in accordance with Nature's laws, they last the lifetime of the animal, and are not subject to disease. Thus we find in animals in their natural state sound teeth to the end of life.

The elephant a hundred years old has no defective teeth, unless they have been injured by accident, or have been made to eat improper food in the service of man. But animals subjected to unnatural food have defective teeth, and, if shorter lived than man, and the enamel less firm, are sooner influenced by improper food.

The teeth of the cow, for example, that is made to live on the dregs of breweries and distilleries, begin to decay in a very short time. But in this case the cause of the decay is not physiological so much as mechanical, for it is found that the decay is more or less rapid according to the temperature of the swill which they are obliged to eat — those at a distance from the distillery, whose food gets cold before it reaches them, preserving their teeth longer than those who, being near, take it hot from the vat.

This brings us to a consideration of the different laws, the disobedience of which is the cause of defective teeth, as it is of all our diseases and sufferings. The universe, and everything in it, whether of mind or matter, from the inorganic atom that can be seen only with a microscope to the mind of the highest archangel, is moved, and changed, and regulated by fixed laws; and while these laws are permitted to act harmoniously, all is well, but disobedience to any one brings its penalties. All suffering and all defects may, therefore, be traced to the disobedience of some law of our being; and the question before us is, Why do not our teeth, like the teeth of other animals, last our lifetime? That they are made as perfect, if the right materials are furnished, there cannot be a doubt.

But are the necessary elements furnished to children as they are to the young of other animals? And do we not subject our teeth to deleterious influences from which animals that obey their natural instincts are exempt?

The forming young of other animals, while dependent on the mother, get lime, and phosphorus, and potash, and silex, and all the other elements of which the teeth are composed, from the blood or milk of the mother, and she gets them from the food which Nature provides containing these elements in their natural proportions.

But where can the child in its forming state get these necessary elements, whose mother lives principally on starch, and butter, and sugar, neither of which contains a particle of lime, phosphorus, potash, or silex? Nature performs no miracles. She makes teeth as glass is made, by combining the elements which compose them according to her own chemical principles. And this illustration is the more forcible, because the composition of the enamel of the teeth and of glass is very nearly identical; both, at least, requiring the combination of silex with some alkaline principle.

If, then, the mother of an unborn or nursing infant lives on white bread and butter, pastry, and confectionery, which contain no silex, and very little of the other elements which compose the teeth, nothing short of a miracle can give her a child with good teeth, and especially with teeth well enamelled.

Nature does what she can for innocent and helpless unborn and nursing infants, by using all available materials, even getting them from the teeth of the mother. And hence, it is well known, that starch, butter, and sugar-eating young mothers always suffer most from their teeth, and go to the dentist most, while an infant is dependent on them for support, as they suffer also, at these times, from neuralgia, headaches, dyspepsia, &c., as I have elsewhere explained, for want of the elements which keep the brain and nerves in a healthy condition.

Thus, instead of "visiting the iniquity of the fathers upon the children," Nature, as far as possible, protects innocent children, and visits on their mothers the penalty for their own transgressions. But there are cases where, in accordance with natural law, children must suffer for the transgressions of their parents. And defective teeth are an illustration of this statement. The enamel of the teeth, wanting, as it is, and from the nature of its composition must be, in all recuperative power, if once broken or defective can never be restored, and the toothache that follows from the inflammation and exposure of the nerves, &c., the child must suffer, while the mother alone is responsible. But this is an exceptional case; all other organs, having recuperative power, are capable of restoration, even though they may be feeble and defective in consequence of the mother's neglect; and even this exception may, by restoring deficient elements, be confined to the first set of teeth. This, being a very important practical point, deserves to be strongly presented.

Second Teeth may be made Sound where the first were Defective.

The second tooth of a child is formed from materials furnished in the blood, secreted, or taken up, and used in forming it by a mysterious power imparted to the little gland, or nucleus, placed for that purpose directly under the first tooth, but entirely independent of it. This mysterious power acts in this, as in all other organs, with unerring certainty, and if the right elements are furnished in the blood, will be sure to find them, and furnish them in right proportions to the forming tooth.

It is, therefore, no more certain that glass can be made by using the right materials in the right way than it is certain that teeth, good and sound, will be made by using the right materials in the right way. Cheer up, then, disconsolate mothers, who weep and mourn, as you must, for the toothache of your little one, for which you feel to be responsible. If the second teeth are yet to come, you have still space for repentance, and works meet for repentance.

But what articles of food will make good teeth? Good milk will make good teeth, for it makes them for calves. Good meat will make good teeth, for it makes them for lions and wolves. Good vegetables and fruits will make good teeth, for they make them for monkeys.

Good corn, oats, barley, wheat, rye, and indeed everything that grows, will make good teeth, if eaten in their natural state, no elements being taken out; for every one of them does make teeth for horses, cows, sheep, or some other animal. But starch, sugar, lard, or butter will not make good teeth. You tried them all with your child's first teeth, and failed; and your neighbors have tried them, and indeed all Christendom has tried them, and the result is that a man or woman at forty with good, sound teeth is a very rare exception.

Nothing, then, can be clearer than your duty to keep from your children confectionery, pastry, white bread and butter, gingerbread and sweet cakes, and feed them instead on milk, unbolted bread, meats, eggs, fruits, vegetables, or anything else in short which they best relish, from which have not been taken any of their native elements. But you must attend to this early; for if children live on carbonaceous food, and the necessary elements are not furnished till the second teeth are formed, "there remaineth no more sacrifice for sin, but a fearful looking for of judgment." The teeth will either come in a defective state, or the enamel will be thin and easily broken, and the juices of the mouth, being admitted into the tooth, cause its decay, without the possibility of cure. For a time, the orifice being filled, the decay may be suspended; but the enamel being imperfect and thin, will soon give way in some other place, and there is no saving them.

Are Sugar and other purely Carbonaceous Food positively injurious to the Teeth, so that they can never be safely taken?

Sugar, starch, butter, lard, &c., contain necessary elements for furnishing animal heat and fat, and no elements directly injurious to the teeth or any other organ; and if we took them only as needed, would never do harm; but furnished, as they are to the requisite extent, in the staple articles of food, as milk, all kinds of grain, meats, &c., and getting as we do from them all that the system requires, the butter, lard, sugar, &c., which we take either combined with one another or with articles of natural food, go to furnish extra fat or heat if digested, and if not digested, — as mostly they are not, — go to produce disorder to the stomach and digestive organs, in passing off in an undigested and fermented state. And this extra food, and these derangements which it produces, prevent the taking enough nitrogenous and phosphatic food to supply the teeth and other organs with their necessary nourishment. (See Philosophy of Eating, page 19.)

They do harm also, undoubtedly, to the teeth by foul secretions which they produce, and which are deposited in sordes or tartar on them; and also by heating the blood, rendering the gums more susceptible to inflammations, and the nerves more susceptible to pain.

But we do not, and we need not always eat such articles as contain a sufficient amount of carbonaceous matter, and therefore need not always abstain from butter, sugar, or fine flour.

If we eat beefsteak, or any other meat, without its natural fat, there is no harm in using, instead, butter, which makes it palatable, and furnishes at the same time a substitute for its natural fat. Most kinds of fish also have not sufficient carbonaceous matter, and especially in winter require fat pork, butter, or lard to furnish heating material. Fruits also contain very little heating matter, but what they do contain is in the form of sugar.

Sugar, therefore, seems to be adapted to them, and may be useful with them, especially if they are too acid to be agreeable. Flour also, or starch in any other form, may be used with cheese, or other concentrated nitrogenous or phosphatic food, especially if the bowels are irritable and cannot bear coarse food, or if some coarse food be eaten at the same meal, to supply the necessary waste. So that, used with discretion, either of these mischief-making carbonaceous articles may be eaten at times with impunity; and in small quantities will never do essential harm, if we are careful to take with them other food in sufficient quantities to supply the necessary elements which they do not contain.

But to attempt to live, and bring up children, on white bread and molasses or butter, cakes, pies, gingerbread, flour, starch, farina, or rice puddings, with sugar, molasses, or butter for sauce, is to starve not only the teeth, but the muscles, bones, all solid tissues, nerves and brains; for there is in neither of these articles but very little food for either.

For a striking illustration of the importance of these suggestions, see a record of experiments on Scottish prisoners (Philosophy of Eating, page 99), and especially notice one fact: The food in Dundee and Edinburgh prisons was exactly the same, except that in Edinburgh milk was eaten with oatmeal porridge and cakes, and in Dundee molasses. At the end of two months the milk-eating prisoners had about one pound each more of flesh than those who ate molasses, and were in much better general condition.

In view of this experiment, and the principle which it illustrates, I induced the matron of an orphan asylum, where the children had been accustomed to eat bread and molasses twice a day, to give them bread and milk instead; and the improvement in their condition was manifest almost immediately.

That there are other predisposing and exciting causes of defective teeth besides extra carbonaceous or deficient phosphatic elements in food, there is no doubt, as I shall presently explain; but the theory is certainly corroborated by observation, that this is the principal cause.

People who live on natural Food have good Teeth, while those who live on extra Carbonaceous Food have bad Teeth.

Savages, whether herbivorous or carnivorous, have good teeth. Our Pilgrim fathers, who ate their grains and their meats as Nature furnished them, with all their requisite elements, had good teeth, as have also the laboring classes of Europe, and indeed of the whole world who live in a similar manner; and if there be a people, or any considerable number of a people, living on natural food, who have much work for dentists, I have not heard of them.

On the other hand, we, the degenerate sons of our healthy and robust Pilgrim fathers, laboring men and all, who make fine flour, butter, sugar, lard, and fat pork our staple articles of food, more generally than any other people in the world, have more work for dentists. And even our Celtic and Hibernian citizens, who come to this country from their diet of oatmeal porridge, barley-cake, cheese and buttermilk, with good teeth at any age, falling into our habits, and using the very finest flour, with butter and lard, and perhaps salt pork, with vegetables swimming in grease, soon begin to lose their teeth, and the teeth of their children are as bad as those of native born citizens of the purest Yankee blood.

We have, then, both from the structure of the teeth, and from collateral evidence, indubitable proof that good teeth are made and kept in repair only with food containing the elements of which good teeth are constructed, of which starch, butter, all oils, and sugar contain not a particle. Of other causes of decay in teeth, that next in importance to want of proper elements, is the irregular temperature to which they are exposed.

Alternation of Heat and Cold a Cause of Decay of Teeth.

To understand this statement, we have but to consider that the enamel of the teeth, which protects the internal parts from decay, and glass are not only alike, as we have explained, in chemical composition, but in density of structure and frangibility. They are also alike under the influence of the physical law of expansion by heat and contraction by cold, and are affected by it as other substances are of the same density and frangibility. If a thin shell of glass, of irregular shape, like the enamel of the teeth, were to be immersed in hot water, and then suddenly into cold, it would crack, probably in many directions, and the continued alternation of heat and cold would, after a while, so open these cracks as to admit through them air and water. And must not the effect on the teeth be the same, exposed as they are at one time to almost boiling hot tea and coffee, and at another to ice-water, or ice-cream — a change of temperature of from seventy-five to one hundred degrees?

If once cracked, and the air and juices of the mouth admitted, there being no remedial power to heal it, decay is inevitable; for though at one decayed point the dentist may, by filling the orifice and excluding the air, water, &c., for a while stop or prolong the process of decay, yet at other weak points the process will still go on, and thus the teeth are lost.

Brushing and cleaning may also retard the process of decay; but brushing with a stiff brush injures the gums, and loosens them from the teeth, to which they ought firmly to adhere, and cleaning with acids hastens the decay, by decomposing the enamel; cleaning with gritty, grinding substances also wears it off; and as most dentifrices are composed of one or the other of these deleterious substances, dentifrices probably, on the whole, do much more harm than good.

Cold water is the best dentifrice, but even that would not be needed if we lived on natural food, as in that case no sordes, or tartar, or any impurities gather on the teeth, the secretions of the mouth being naturally pure as the purest water. And this is shown by the fact that animals which live on natural food have mouths and teeth perfectly clean, without the use of brushes and dentifrices; and that these devices are not needed to preserve sound teeth is also shown by the same fact.

Elephants preserve their teeth a hundred years, — some say five hundred, — without the use of either tooth-brush or dentifrice, and the tooth of the elephant is composed of precisely the same elements as the tooth of man, while the teeth of man begin to decay in infancy, and are in a sound state on an average probably not more than ten years.

An explanation of this difference will, I think, corroborate my view of the cause of defective teeth, and sum up the whole matter.

Elephants live always on natural food, and always therefore get all the elements necessary for making good teeth, and for keeping them in health, and of course baby elephants, having these elements while dependent on the mother, commence life with perfect teeth, and are never afterwards without means of preserving them. Mothers of infant children, living as they do in New England, and in all American and European cities, cannot furnish their dependent children with the necessary elements for making good teeth; and children, following in the habits of their mothers, never get the right materials for keeping their teeth in repair.

Again; elephants, always taking their food at nearly the same temperature, never expose their teeth to changes that crack the enamel and cause them to decay; while men and women, and sometimes even children, between their tea and their ice-water, which they sometimes take at the same meal, subject them to a change of one hundred degrees within the space of fifteen, and sometimes even five minutes.

Are Defective Teeth hereditary?

Some of the phenomena of hereditary diseases and deformities are very mysterious and very curious. Brown-Sequard, in a very interesting lecture on Epilepsy, which I attended, mentioned a fact which illustrates this statement. While in the hospital in London for the treatment of epilepsy, he experimented on different animals with a view to determine the cause of that disease, and he found that on many animals he could always induce epilepsy by irritating the spinal marrow at the base of the skull. These animals would afterwards be subject to epilepsy; and Guinea pigs, which were never known to have that disease, except after such an operation, would not only have it afterwards, but their offspring would also have it, showing that diseases *can be inherited that were induced by accident or injury.*

I know two children, in whom the first joint of the little finger on the left hand stands at right angles with the other joints. Their father, before he was married, had the little finger on the same hand put out of joint, and it was never set. I know also a young lady who, when particularly interested in anything, looks at it aslant; and this was the peculiarity of her mother, whom she never saw after she was six weeks old: but it was the peculiarity of the maternal ancestry for five or six generations, one or two in a family only having it. And having been traced to a family by the name of Green, it is familiarly known among all the relations as the "Green squint."

I knew also a young man, whose father died when he was an infant, who always reminded his friends of his father by a peculiar shrug of the shoulders and a peculiar gait.

For such congenital peculiarities there is no explanation, and they are recorded only as constitutional curiosities. But there is a class of hereditary diseases, to which I think those of the teeth belong, which are more explicable, and the consideration of which is of much greater practical importance — such as are transmitted to children by transmitting the wrong habits which produced them. Such can be warded off in all cases and cured in all cases, except those of the teeth, which have no recuperative power, by changing those wrong habits for right ones. An example of this we have seen in the chapter on Apoplexy, where strong hereditary tendencies were warded off, and even the symptoms of it removed, by appropriate diet and regimen.

What we inherit of diseases and imperfections of the teeth is merely the want of elements necessary for good sound teeth; and from the peculiar construction of them, these diseases and imperfections can never be restored, as I have before explained. But by supplying right elements, the next generation may be secured from defective teeth, and even the present generation, as has been explained, if the second teeth are not yet formed.

I have seen a mother consoling herself for the defective teeth of her child, on the ground that her own teeth were bad, and her mother's before her, and therefore bad teeth must be inevitable in her family. The fact is, she lived on carbonaceous food, and drank hot tea, and the consequences were inevitable. If her child lives on natural food, and avoids other causes of defective teeth, the consequences will be also inevitable, and the next generation will begin with good teeth; and by continuing the course, will continue to have good teeth, and they will be transmitted from generation to generation.

HOW TO PREVENT DISEASES OF HEART.

THE circulation of the blood is a mechanical operation, and the action of the heart on the blood, drawing it from every part of the system through the veins, and sending it to every part through the arteries, is like the action of a fire-engine drawing water from a cistern through a hose, and sending it, at the same time, through another hose, into every part of a building on fire. And the arrangement of valves by which this double action is accomplished is alike in both operations.

Many of the difficulties and embarrassments of the action of the heart are also mechanical. Sometimes there is an organic congenital malformation by which the heart is imperfect, and, of course, it can never perfectly perform its function, and the circulation is irregular and defective. Sometimes the valves get out of order, or become hardened like bone, and act very imperfectly in preventing the regurgitation of blood, and, of course, the circulation is deranged. Sometimes the accumulation of fat around the heart prevents its free expansion, and embarrasses its action. Sometimes contraction of the chest, as in tight dressing, embarrasses the action of the heart, and palpitation and fainting are produced; and this, indeed, is so commonly the cause of fainting that everybody almost instinctively cuts the strings at once, in such cases, as a rational means of relief.

Sometimes the embarrassment is from increased pressure of the blood, causing distention of the blood-vessels and of the heart. Sometimes the embarrassment and irregular action are caused by irritability of the nervous system, and sometimes by overheated and stimulating blood. We may not be able perfectly to understand the cause of all these different difficulties or diseases of the heart; but they are all undoubtedly connected with erroneous diet or erroneous habits, for other animals in their native conditions have none of these troubles or diseases, although the circulation is effected by the same mechanical arrangement.

How congenital defects, or ossification of the valves are produced, I do not profess to understand; but the cause and means of preventing and curing, or, at least, alleviating the other difficulties, I think can be understood and explained.

As we cannot stop the heart, to repair its valves when once deranged, as we can stop an engine for repairs; and as Nature cannot, in the nature of the case, repair ossified or displaced valves, that trouble can never be removed, when once established. And this is true of enlargement of the heart, or arteries, or veins about the heart, or indeed of any other organic affection. And in such cases the question to be considered is, How can such persons live, so as to be comfortable, with such difficulties? The right course of treatment in such cases can be illustrated and enforced, perhaps, by the management and results of two cases.

More than thirty years ago I was consulted in two cases of organic diseases of the heart very nearly alike, and very clear cases of incurable disease. Both of about the same age, free livers, and accustomed to stimulating food and some stimulating drinks, but of very different tempers; of religious character, and power of self-control, and both so seriously affected as frequently, when excited or fatigued, to fall into an unconscious state, and remain in it for hours. They were both told their lives were in their own hands, and advised to abstain from carbonaceous food, stimulating drinks, condiments, and medicines; avoid all excitements, mental and physical, and never allow themselves to run or get fatigued, even if their houses should burn down over their heads — in that case just deliberately walk out and let them burn, rather than fight the fire themselves.

Their reception of the advice was characteristic of the two men, and the results such as might have been expected. One said, after a few moments of silence, but in great agitation, "About dying, I am not particular; but while I do live I shall have my brandy and my fat beef as usual. I am not to be all my lifetime subject to bondage for fear of death." — In less than three weeks some neighbors' hogs got into his garden, just as he had finished his dinner of fat beef, and had taken his brandy to make it digest. In great excitement he ran out after them, and fell down dead in the garden.

The other gentleman said, "It is clearly my duty to 'keep under my body, and bring it into subjection,' according to the example of the Apostle." — He is now living, at the age of seventy-six, and enjoying comfortable health, having, for thirty years, lived "a quiet and peaceable life, in all godliness and honesty," and having been exempt from those fainting fits which so distressed and alarmed his friends; indeed, having enjoyed vastly more in eating and drinking than if he had put no restraints on his appetites, and even more than if he had only put on them such restraints as are customary in the class of virtuous and excellent people to which he belongs.

If palpitation, shortness of breath on going up stairs, fainting fits, distress about the heart, any or all are produced, as they often are in persons predisposed to obesity, by accumulation of fat about the heart, the remedy is simple and sure: for if the material of which fat is made be not supplied, fat will not only not be made, but if made will be absorbed. Follow, therefore, the directions given in the chapter on Corpulence.

If these symptoms are produced by tight lacing, the remedy is equally simple, and upon the same principle — stop the supply of strings, and belts, and corsets.

If they are produced by heating food, stimulating drinks and condiments, of course these are also to be withdrawn, and the cure is certain. If by derangement of the nervous system, follow the directions in the chapter on Apoplexy, Neuralgia, and Nervous Diseases.

While, therefore, I do not deny that there are cases of enlargement of the heart and arteries that must prove fatal in spite of all treatment, yet, in most cases, by following the foregoing suggestions, I have not a doubt that in functional cases a radical cure can be effected, and in organic, a great modification and improvement of the symptoms.

HOW TO CURE CORPULENCE.

Adipose substance, or fat, is deposited under the skin for three purposes: 1. To protect the system from cold, or, in other words, to retain the heat of the body, fat being a good non-conductor of heat. 2. To form an insensible cushion to protect the internal organs from the effects of concussions, pressures, &c. 3. To fill up the angles and interstices formed by the attachments of muscles to the prominences of bone, &c., so as to leave the outlines of the body rounded and beautiful, Nature's lines of beauty being always curved, while sharp and angular lines are given for utility.

This fat is composed of the same carbonaceous elements as are used by the lungs to furnish animal heat, and, if not otherwise supplied, as in case of sickness, when fat or other carbonaceous food cannot be digested, or in fasting, they are supplied by absorbing this adipose covering, and this we call losing flesh, or growing poor.

On this account fat men bear fasting longer than lean men; and on this principle hibernating animals, as the raccoon, badger, and the brown bear, fat up in the summer on the abundance of food that is then furnished them, and in winter crawl into their dens and live on themselves, coming out in the spring poor and haggard, and ready for a new supply. And here we have the foundation for philosophical cure for obesity.

Butter, the fat of meats, starch, and sugar furnish animal heat, and also the adipose covering which, in excess, constitutes corpulence. Some of these principles the lungs must have every moment, or we die for want of animal heat. If, therefore, these carbonaceous principles are not supplied in food, they are taken from the fatty accumulations under the skin — the deposits being withdrawn in case of necessity, just as a banker uses his surplus funds when he gets into a pinch. This withdrawal of fatty deposits is seen every day in fevers and other diseases, when food cannot be digested, and is seen also in fastings, as in shipwrecked mariners, &c.; and it has been proved in such cases that fat men live longer than lean ones.

By experiments on prisoners (see Philosophy of Eating, page 98), it is seen that fourteen ounces of carbonaceous food are required, in a moderate temperature, at rest, to keep up the weight of the body, and by the rations of English soldiers, &c., it is also seen that in active service from twenty to twenty-two ounces are necessary. If less than these amounts are supplied, the balance is withdrawn from the deposits under the skin, as has been proved over and over again by experiment.

The five hundred prisoners, in five different jails in Scotland, above referred to, had, on an average, thirteen ounces each day for two months, and they lost in weight six hundred and fifty-three pounds, varying somewhat in different prisons, according to the different nutritive value of the different articles used; but in like circumstances losing in just the proportion as the sugar, starch, or fat fell below the requisite amount.

We have, then, a standard by which to judge of the requisite amount of starch or sugar necessary to keep the deposit of fat good. We must, however, bear in mind the fact, stated in Philosophy of Eating, page 123, that butter and the fat of all meats contain two and one half times as much fattening qualities, in a given weight, as starch or sugar, containing, as they all do, no water, while starch and sugar contain seventy-five per cent. of water.

If, then, a man of average weight, say one hundred and fifty pounds, wishes to retain the deposits as they now are, and continue that weight, in, perhaps, nineteen cases in twenty he will succeed, and remain, year after year, by eating any of the articles in the foregoing table in such proportions as to get, with his necessary nitrates, from fourteen to twenty-one ounces of carbonates, according to his exercise, in moderate weather — in hot weather less, and in cold weather more.

But it is not expected, nor is it desirable, that he should weigh out his food, and the table is not prepared for that purpose; still it will be found useful to have in mind the relative value of different articles of food in heating and nutritive properties, both while furnishing and eating his dinners.

If he lives on articles of food as Nature has furnished

them, his appetite will direct him both in regard to the quantity to be eaten, and the articles to be eaten together; but, as I have elsewhere explained, if he add to these articles of food either fine flour, which is mostly starch, or sugar, he will, in proportion to the amount used, increase the amount of heating and fattening food without increasing the strengthening; and if he add butter, or lard, or the fat of meats, he adds, in proportion to the amount used, two and one half times as much to his carbonates, without increasing his nitrates.

In that case one of two undesirable consequences will follow — he will increase in fatness, if predisposed to obesity, and the blood will become heated by this extra carbon circulating in it before being deposited, and also by retaining the heat in the system as a non-conductor, or the extra carbonaceous material will be cast off as unnatural waste, and being unnatural will ferment, causing flatulence, and irritation, and the colics, and bowel complaints, which are the natural consequence.

If, on the other hand, he takes food containing less than from fourteen to twenty-one ounces of fat and heat-producing food, he will draw on his deposits to an amount proportionate to the deficiency, and to the amount of exercise which he takes. Moreover, inasmuch as corpulence, or extra fatty deposits, comes generally from extra, and not from natural, carbonaceous food, it is not necessary, except where the constitutional tendency to obesity is very strong, to reduce the supply of natural food at all, as the cause is removed by cutting off the extra carbon, and the extra fat is absorbed.

And, besides, in cases where the tendency to corpulence is not constitutionally strong, it is often only necessary to abstain from that one principle of carbonaceous food which has the strongest tendency to produce fat — doing it, not by the process of digestion, but by a mere transfer of fat from one animal to another, whereas sugar has to be digested to be converted into fat, and starch has first to be converted into sugar before it can be converted into fat.

Of this very simple process of curing obesity, let me give an illustration. A gentleman of ordinary height, who weighed two hundred and ten pounds, and his wife, rather short in stature, who weighed, I think, one hundred and sixty pounds, under my direction tried the experiment of abstaining from butter, and mostly from the fat of all meats, except as they were necessary with steak, fish, &c., which were deficient in this principle; but eating sugar and fine flour moderately, as usual; never, however, using butter with white bread or other farinaceous food, but eating cheese instead.

In a few months the gentleman had withdrawn twenty-five pounds of fatty deposits, and the lady about fifteen. And, being satisfied with their improvement, they have, for the last three years, remained at the same weight, by simply being careful not to eat an excess of any carbonaceous food; eating, however, butter and all kinds of fat within the limits prescribed.

William Banting, the Englishman, is also an example of cure of obesity by abstaining only partially from extra carbonaceous food. He reduced himself, according to the statement in his pamphlet, from two hundred and two to one hundred and fifty-six pounds, by "abstaining as much as possible from bread, butter, milk, sugar, beer, potatoes, and some kinds of wines, as port; and living on beef, mutton, and other meats except pork, and any vegetables except potatoes, with good Madeira, claret, and sherry wines, and a *tumbler of gin, whiskey, or brandy grog, at night*, as a night-cap."

But neither Banting nor his medical adviser seems to have had but an inkling of the principle upon which the change was effected, the one seeming to think it was a process by which to kill a disease which he absurdly calls a "parasite," and the other that it was produced by some chemical effect on the secretions of the liver; but neither comprehended the simple principle on which the whole effect was produced.

Nor did they understand what principles in food should be avoided, or why they should be avoided. Accordingly we find bread, milk, and potatoes condemned, while alcohol and fat meat are allowed. Indeed, the cure seems to have been effected by a mere blunder, in which it happened that, although the alcohol and the fat in beef and mutton must have retarded the process of absorption, and, of course, delayed the cure, still, in spite of this error, the cure in his case was effected by abstaining from starch, sugar, and fat in other food, which brought the amount used daily below the fourteen to twenty ounces required to keep up the deposits. But in the directions given in the pamphlet there is nothing to show that the tumbler of gin, whiskey, or brandy "nightcap" was not as important in the cure as beefsteak or fish; and hundreds who never drank these death-dealing articles before, are now taking, by the recommendation of Banting, enough every night to give them a regular fuddle, as a part of the necessary process of curing obesity. And yet everybody knows that alcohol, in any form, tends to produce obesity — not, however, by adding to the fat, but by retarding absorption.

In spite of these absurd and conflicting recommendations, those whose tendency to corpulence is not very strong, have succeeded in reducing it by these conflicting directions; but, on the other hand, those whose predispositions to it are strong, and whose appetites for carbonaceous food are also strong, fail altogether, or, if they partially succeed, finding the sacrifice too great, fall back to their old habits, and take on again their old burdens of flesh.

But those who set about this matter scientifically, and, instead of confining themselves exclusively to "beef and other meats except pork, any vegetables except potatoes, with good Madeira, claret, and sherry wines, and a tumbler of gin, whiskey, or brandy grog, as a nightcap," and thus being obliged to be more scrupulously abstemious in some things, on account of the counteracting influence of the others, taking from the whole bill of fare which God has given them, consisting of "every living that moveth," and every thing that grows, that is, or can be made, agreeable to the palate in its natural state, or by adding such principles, in an agreeable form, as are needed to supply necessary elements, may eat what they please, and all they desire, and still reduce their surplus fat, if they will only see to it that the carbonaceous matter comes below the requisite fourteen to twenty ounces.

Or the same thing can be accomplished by being careful that no article of food contains more than its due proportion of carbonaceous food, and some contain less; and if some do contain more, that others containing less be used at the same time. For example: Suppose the meal before you consisted of unbolted bread, milk, eggs, beef or mutton, of average fatness, cooked in its own gravy. As all these articles contain just their natural proportions of carbonaceous nourishment, you might eat as much of either or all as the appetite demanded, without increasing your deposits of fat; and if the beef or mutton were perfectly lean, you could add an equivalent for the fat in butter, without varying the effect. But if, instead of unbolted meal bread, your bread was from superfine flour, and instead of milk you had butter, thus far you would get nothing but carbonaceous food; and then if you add to your eggs butter, and to your beef and mutton gravy from fat pork, or flour and butter, you have before you, instead of food containing its natural proportions of carbonates and nitrates, probably double the necessary amount of carbonates; and in eating all you want, to get the necessary supply of muscle-making food, you have eaten, perhaps, a third more fat-making food than is needed, and the surplus must either be added to your adipose deposits, or be thrown off as waste.

Now, this is just what the better classes in England, and all classes in New England, are doing every day; and therefore all who are predisposed to obesity, and have not exercise enough to work it off, are constantly waxing fat, while the lean ones are suffering from the effects of this heating food in some other way.

These facts and these principles cannot be disproved, and it follows that, with but little sacrifice, most people, even if inclined to corpulence, can regulate their weight as they please. Indeed there is not only no sacrifice even of the pleasures of eating, but a positive addition to gustatory pleasures, in confining ourselves to such articles of food as are best adapted to our condition. And this is the testimony of every man who has had perseverance enough to overcome the first cravings of a perverted appetite. After the first short struggle with it, unless the struggle is prolonged by an occasional indulgence, which, of course, prolongs the struggle, the appetite and taste soon conform to their primitive condition of craving and relishing best just the food that is best for us, and we return to our simple, child-like love for natural food, cooked without abstracting any of its essential elements, or adding anything injurious.

LEANNESS: ITS CAUSE AND ITS CURE.

All animals but man are fat or lean as they are fed on carbonaceous food and are kept still, or on nitrogenous food and are permitted to run at large. The farmer lets his oxen run at large, or works them, till the muscles are developed, and they are grown to a sufficient size to be profitable for beef, and then shuts them up, and feeds them freely on Indian corn meal, and they immediately begin to fatten up for beef, and within certain limits the fat accumulates in proportion to the meal they can be induced to eat.

In some places, also, hogs are permitted to range in woods and fields for acorns and grass till they are sufficiently grown, and then are brought in, as poor as hounds, to be fatted up for the market; and a calculation can be made with accuracy as to how many pounds they are gaining each week, by noticing how much corn meal is consumed; and two pigs of the same family will generally keep of about the same weight if treated in the same way.

But let a family of men live on the same food, and have the same amount of exercise and the same general habits, and some members will be lean as wolves, and others as fat as pigs.

The same elements are found to compose the flesh of the pig as compose the flesh of man, and the same general arrangements are found for digestion and assimilation, and generally, especially in their fully domesticated state, the same kinds of food are given to them as to men. Pigs, however, get the skimmed milk and bran, which strengthen the powers of digestion, while men get the butter and fine flour, which weaken the powers of digestion; and this fact gives us the means of explaining the otherwise enigmatical question, —

Why is it that a pig, with digestive organs and appetites, if not habits and dispositions, like his master, should always, with good food, be "fat and flourishing," while his master, with better, or at least more carbonaceous food, may be as "ill-favored and lean-fleshed" as Pharaoh's kine? Let us see if this enigma can be explained.

We are fattened, as we are strengthened, not necessarily by what we eat, but by what we digest; and constantly overburdened as the human stomach is (in this country among all classes, and in the cities of Europe among the better classes) with an excess of carbonaceous food, such as butter, sugar, lard, starch, &c., which is never all digested, after a while it seems to get discouraged and to cease to try to digest it.

In such cases, those who are predisposed to obesity become fat, but weak, languid, and stupid, — the carbonaceous food being better digested than the nitrogenous or phosphatic; while those who are predisposed to leanness may have muscular or mental strength, — the nitrogenous and phosphatic in them being digested, but not the carbonaceous, — but become lean and haggard, and the redundant carbonaceous food, except that which supplies animal heat, is all wasted, and that, in such persons, is generally deficient.

But pigs, not having predispositions, except to obesity, and not often having their digestive powers weakened or embarrassed by extra carbonaceous food, digest and give credit for all they eat. I have been told, however, that pigs may be cloyed by overfeeding, so as to lose flesh while more corn meal is before them than they can eat, and that, by continued overfeeding, they will continue to grow lean. In such cases, in order to fatten them, the food must first be withheld until they become hungry, and then, by feeding at first sparingly, and keeping the supply below the demand, their digestive powers will gradually recover, and they will fatten like other pigs.

Here, then, we have an illustration of my position as to the cause of leanness, and at the same time a hint as to the cure of it. The cause of leanness, in this country at least, is never the want of carbonaceous food, but from overloading the stomach with it, as before described. What, then, can be more rational than to take a hint from the farmer with his pigs, and keep the stomach supplied with good strengthening and fattening food only just as it is really wanted and will be digested, never eating without an appetite, and never eating anything but good food, so cooked and served as to be eaten with a good relish?

In this way, I venture to assert, that any man, however predisposed to leanness, may give his bones an adipose covering to any desirable extent. But what course will secure perpetually a good appetite, a good relish for food, and good digestion?

How to secure a good Appetite.

A good appetite cannot be permanently secured without regularity in times of eating.

The stomach cannot, like the heart and lungs, work continually, but is intended to have its time for labor and its time for rest. It is, however, very accommodating, and will furnish the requisite juices, and perform the requisite labor of digesting food, once, twice, and even four or five times a day, if its task is given it at regular hours; but it must have rest: and to insure vigorous digestion, that rest must be as long and continuous as the regular hours of sleep. The frequency and time of meals for laboring men, — if they can have good nourishing food, and that which is not too easily digested, — are probably three times in twenty-four hours, say at six in the morning, twelve at noon, and six at night, the morning and noon meals containing the principal elements for muscular power, while the evening meal is such as will not, in the exhausted state of the system, require much digestive labor. And for sedentary men two meals are sufficient — one in the morning and one in the afternoon, at some regular hour. With this arrangement a good appetite will be secured at every meal, especially if we scrupulously avoid taking food between meals, or within three hours of the regular time for sleep. Digestion will go on while we sleep, unless the powers of the system are greatly exhausted by the labors of the day; but sleep is never quiet and refreshing while the stomach is oppressed with food, and digestion is never well done while the system is exhausted, as we have all had occasion to notice.

And here, perhaps, as well as elsewhere, I may explain the reason for these suggestions. Sleep — "tired Nature's sweet restorer" — imparts to the system all the nervous or vital energy which is necessary for the duties of the day, and to keep all our functions in healthy, harmonious action, and secure a good appetite for food. This vital energy must be expanded during waking hours, partly in mental, partly in muscular, and partly in digestive exercise. We may so expend it all in intense and continuous mental effort as to have none left for muscular or digestive powers, as we have seen in cases where lawyers or legislators have given their whole powers of mind to an important case till Nature became exhausted, and they could neither walk nor digest food till partially restored by sleep. Or we may so expend the vital energy in muscular exertion as to exhaust the whole vital force, and not be able to think or to digest food till the vital energy is restored by sleep. Of this we have seen examples in men at a fire, or in a flood, or some other similar emergency, who would fall down in utter exhaustion; and to prevent taxing the digestive powers in such a state, Nature provides that all food should be thrown from the stomach, and none afterwards received till sleep should restore the exhausted powers. Or we may so engorge the stomach as to expend all our vital powers on digestion, and become incapable of mental and physical exercise, and even to destroy the powers of life. Of this we have seen frequent examples. Two miserable men made a wager on eating eggs. The man who should eat the greatest number in twelve hours should be supplied with grog for a week. Before the end of twelve hours both fell into a stertorous sleep, from which one never recovered, and the other not for some days.

From these principles and facts we get some valuable hints in regard to mental, physical, and digestive management, and may infer that if we desire a good appetite in the morning, when, having most vital power, a good appetite is most valuable, we must not eat a hearty meal at night, when the system is exhausted, but must always give the stomach its regular tasks and its time to rest; and this is found to be true in other animals whose digestive apparatus is like that of men.

The horse is kept in good condition only by being fed at regular times, and pigs also thrive much better if food is withheld except at regular hours.

To secure a good appetite we must eat good food.

Food, to be perfectly digested, as we have elsewhere seen, must be taken only in such quantities as the system demands, and if we take only natural food, in which is the appropriate mixture of necessary elements, the appetite can always be trusted to interpret the demands of the system, and in that case we should never eat too much. But eating, as we do, flour, butter, and sugar, which have but a part of the elements required, these articles can only be digested as they are eaten with food deficient in the elements which they contain, and these are very few. Consequently these redundant articles, in just about the proportions in which they are eaten, remain undigested in the stomach and bowels, causing flatulence and derangement of the secretions of the stomach, mouth, and all the digestive organs, and the sordes of the teeth, bad taste in the mouth, foulness of breath, and fastidious appetite, &c., which they always have who live on these concentrated carbonaceous articles.

I have often wished — but of course never dared to suggest the idea — that our fastidious, confectionery and cake-eating young ladies, who have no appetite except for unnatural carbonaceous food, and whose breath in consequence is so offensive to themselves as to require constantly some aromatic seeds or some patent trix, and whose mouth is so filled with offensive saliva, and whose teeth so covered with sordes, that charcoal and a tooth-brush used every day will not keep them clean, might look into the mouth of a cow, a dog, or even a pig, neither of which use charcoal, tooth-brush, or trix, and see how clean the mouth and teeth are, and how pure the secretions, and — ("angels and ministers of grace defend me!") — *how sweet their breath is!* — comparatively. Now why is not the breath of a young lady as sweet as that of a —— little child, who needs no more charcoal, trix, or tooth-brush than a pig? and why is not her appetite always as good, and her teeth as clean? No reason can be given but that to which I have referred. Little children, cows, dogs, and pigs digest all their food, and the waste passes off, leaving the system pure. The food of the young lady who eats cakes, pastry, starch, and butter, remains undigested, to derange all the digestive functions and secretions in just the proportion as these carbonaceous articles take the place of natural food.

That this is not a mere theory, can be proved by looking into the mouth of any young lady who carefully avoids all extra carbonaceous food; and such young ladies are now frequently met, and I thank God for the belief that the number is rapidly increasing. Such ladies need no charcoal or trix to neutralize or disguise the impurity of secretions, or to correct an offensive breath, and no brush to keep the teeth clean; and if, in other respects, their habits are good and regular, they always have a good appetite at meal time.

How to secure good Relish for Food.

The importance of eating food with a good relish we have elsewhere explained (see Philosophy of Eating, pages 213–218, also the chapter on Dyspepsia); and we have also shown what considerations are necessary in regard to cooking, condiments, &c.

What we now want to know is, what course will best

secure such a relish for every meal of food as to induce digestion sufficient to supply the wastes of the system, and have a surplus for filling up the sharp angles, and for covering up the bones and muscles with a warm and comely coat, and to secure this influence permanently, according to the evident intention of Nature? For a single meal, that which combines a good supply of carbonaceous elements with nitrogenous and phosphatic, in such a manner and with such accompaniments as to secure the highest possible gustatory enjoyments, would be most fattening; but extraordinary gustatory enjoyments can no more be permanent than other extraordinary pleasures, and the reaction and subsequent disrelish for common and natural enjoyments are proportionate to the excess. And to attempt to keep up the relish for food by keeping up a supply of everything especially agreeable, would prove an utter failure; for they enjoy the least who try the hardest to tempt the appetite with the greatest variety of good things. Soon becoming cloyed with everything rich and savory, while nothing else can be relished, the choicest viands, however nicely prepared, become loathsome and even disgusting.

But the appetite never cloys with food as Nature furnishes it, if so prepared as best to develop the relish which naturally belongs to it, especially if we cook but a small variety for the same meal, so that some variety can be had continually; but if we cook together to-day all the variety of meats and vegetables in common use, and mingle their flavor together, as is done in restaurants and hotels, although we may have for once an agreeable combination of flavors, yet having, as we must have, the same combination to-morrow, the next day, and continually, it soon becomes tiresome.

To secure good digestion and a good adipose covering, two things more are needed, — one is to eat slowly, and the other is included in that beautiful description of a good and happy people, they "did eat their meat with gladness and singleness of heart."

Good Digestion depends on eating deliberately.

No one habit in this country contributes so largely to dyspepsia and leanness as that of bolting food. Probably the average length of time devoted to the principal meals is not over fifteen minutes among business men, mechanics, and laborers. That such a habit must be productive of indigestion, and consequent leanness, will be made apparent by considering the object accomplished by masticating food. One great object is to keep in the mouth, in contact with the nerves of taste, the savory morsel till its flavor has aroused the secretions of the juices, which are the principal agents in the process of digestion, and gathered them not only in the mouth, but also in the stomach. That the presence in the mouth, and even the sight and smell of food which we relish, does arouse these secretions, we cannot have failed to notice.

Another object in masticating food is so to comminute it, that when received into the stomach the gastric juice will be admitted at once to every particle, and the process of digestion be commenced at once in every part of the morsel. But how different from this natural condition is the food in the stomach of the man who bolts his food in morsels as large as can be made to pass down, and, in the time necessary to prepare a single ounce for easy digestion, has filled his capacious maw with these enormous masses of indigestible food! I have seen masses of beef thrown from the stomach after remaining there undigested three or four days, or even a week.

Can we wonder, then, that we find among our merchants and business men, who never can spare but fifteen minutes for their meals, so many cadaverous, desiccated, "ill-favored and lean-fleshed" specimens of humanity? The wonder is, that, not conforming to the conditions on which good healthy juices are secreted, and not comminuting the food, so that those that are formed can come in contact with the massive morsels, except on their surface, enough can be digested to keep them alive.

Good Digestion is promoted by Cheerfulness.

Nothing is better understood than that there is a connection between cheerfulness and good digestion; and the trite expression, "to laugh and grow fat," undoubtedly had its origin in observation, if not in philosophy. What an astonishing amount and variety of food can be disposed of, and perfectly digested, at one sitting of two or three hours, by a company of cheerful and happy, not to say jolly and merry, old friends, and that without alcohol, or any other unnatural stimulus, to help digestion! I venture to say more than three times as much as the same individuals could eat and digest in the same time if each took his meals by himself.

And this one fact is worth more than all else I can write to show the dependence of the digestive powers on the state of the mind, and to prove that he must be lean and haggard who, keeping his mind constantly on his business, bolts his meals in silence and solitude, even in the presence of his family. I commend it to the careful consideration of uncomfortable mortals who never properly digest their food, and whose bones are too poorly clothed with flesh, and too poorly protected ever to allow them quiet rest, and who, therefore, envy "fat, sleek-headed men, and such as sleep o' nights."

From these considerations I venture to affirm, that any man not absolutely sick, who so trusts in Providence as to be able to obey the spirit of the injunction, "Take no thought for the morrow;" who keeps from his stomach, except as they are needed for animal heat, such heating food as butter, starch, and sugar, and who, therefore, digests all he eats; who eats at such regular and appropriate times as to secure rest for the stomach and a good appetite; who never taxes the stomach with food when tired and exhausted; who eats nothing that cannot be relished, and nothing the relish of which is not natural, or allows anything to enter the stomach that is not needed as food or drink; who takes his food so deliberately as to have it properly masticated and lubricated, and who eats his "meat with gladness and singleness of heart," will be exempt from dyspepsia, and his bones will be covered with a comfortable and comely coating of flesh.

MEDICINES: THEIR USES AND ABUSES.

MEDICINES are undoubtedly a gift from God, intended to relieve suffering, and assist Nature in the cure of disease. This is a fair inference, from the fact that some medicines certainly do, under some circumstances, relieve pain, and do assist Nature in the cure of disease; and whatever good in Nature anything can do for man it was undoubtedly intended to do, the world being understood to be made for man, and everything in it intended to subserve his interests. But it is universally admitted that medicines, as they have been and still are generally used, do also much harm; indeed, it is the opinion of the best physicians that

Medicines have always done much more Harm than Good.

Sir Astley Cooper, the most celebrated English practitioner of the last generation, has left on record his opinion, that, on the whole, more harm than good is done by medication.

Dr. Worthington Hooker, of New Haven, in his prize essay, published in 1857, says he believes that the peculiar form of typhus fever which prevailed some years ago in New England, and which, being treated with stimulants, was very fatal, "was often, in fact, a brandy and opium disease."

Dr. O. W. Holmes, in his address of May 30, 1860, makes this admission to the Massachusetts Medical Society: "Throw out opium, throw out a few specifics which our art did not discover, throw out wine, and the vapors which produce the miracle of anæsthesia, and I firmly believe that if the whole *materia medica*, as now used, could be sunk to the bottom of the sea, it would be all the better for mankind, and all the worse for the fishes."

Now, no one who believes the Bible will affirm that these are the legitimate effects of medicine, for the record is that "God saw everything that he had made, and behold it was very good." If this be a true record, there must be something wrong in the dogma of what is called "rational medicine," which is so often quoted by the leading men of that school, and so ludicrously referred to in the foregoing quotation from Dr. Holmes.

"Drugs, in themselves considered, may always be regarded as Evils," a false idea.

This idea is not consistent with their own belief in regard to the effects of some medicines, for four or five drugs are known to rational practitioners under the name of alteratives, or specifics, "to produce a secret change in the system favorable to recovery from disease," and this in doses so small as to be tasteless, and to produce no perceptible evils; and hundreds are equally well known, to new school practitioners, to produce similar effects. And is it reasonable to suppose that other drugs are intended by Nature to effect a cure only by producing such serious evils as to make it a question whether the effects of the medicine or the effects of the disease are most to be feared? Is it not more "rational" to suppose that drugs, like every other blessing from God, are intended for good, and for good only, and that the wrong application of them produces the evils which are known to result from them? For illustration: in testing my old school drugs in my new school practice, — and this is the best use to which I can apply my knowledge of crude drugs, — I find constant corroborations of this belief.

In using rhubarb, or calomel, for example, as I often did in operative doses, for the cure of diarrhœa, the patient was reduced and his digestive functions were deranged, but the disease was cured; and, until I learned the truth, I was reconciled to the evils on account of the benefits of the medicine. But I now find rhubarb or calomel much more useful in the same disease, in doses too small to reduce the patient or derange his digestive functions; and the inference, to my mind, is fair, that in large doses the cure was effected in spite of the active operation, and not on account of it. I have tested many medicines in the same way, with this uniform result: where large doses of medicine will cure a disease, with accompanying evils, small doses will accomplish the same end without such evils.

And yet, so universal is the opinion that medicine can do no good except in a form in which it is capable of doing harm, that we meet this argument against diluted medicine everywhere. "I knew of a child that swallowed a whole bottleful, and it did him no harm," and this is supposed to settle all controversy on this subject.

Surely such doctrines as these came neither from the "book of Nature," nor from the "book of Grace," for in these nothing can be found to correspond with this idea of doing "evil that good may come." They came from an age when the light of Nature had shone but very dimly, and when the light of the gospel had not yet dawned upon the world.

Hippocrates, the acknowledged father of "rational practice," who wrote three hundred years before the Christian era, expressed so very exactly the sentiments of Professor Holmes, in his "Currents and Counter Currents in Medical Science," from which the foregoing quotation was taken, as to form, at least, a wonderful coincidence, the only discoverable difference being this: Hippocrates, "lest Nature might be disturbed in her wholesome operation on the matter of disease," never, in any case, gave medicine till after the most active symptoms had subsided, while the professor does make an exception in favor of three or four diseases which the specifics are adapted to cure. The improvement in rational practice in two thousand years amounts, then, to simply this: A specific has been discovered for the itch, for syphilis, and for intermittent fever, and possibly for some two or three other diseases — but they are not named by the professor. Except the medicines adapted to cure these interesting diseases, so wonderfully favored by Nature, the professor firmly believes "that if the whole *materia medica, as now used*, could be sunk to the bottom of the sea, it would be all the better for mankind, and all the worse for the fishes." He does offer to "throw out" wine and opium, which Hippocrates undoubtedly used, and the anæsthetic vapors, which, though not understood to cure disease, are undoubtedly a great blessing to mankind.

This, then, is the condition of rational medicine in the middle of the nineteenth century. There are known to be thousands of varieties of diseases, and thousands of varieties of medicines; and a few of these diseases have medicines adapted to their cure; but all the rest of the diseases are to be trusted to Nature for cure, and all the rest of the medicines are to be thrown into the sea, as worse than useless. But have we not here a marvellous exception to the uniformity of Nature's laws?

We never find an eye where there is not light to act upon it. And so uniform is this law that fishes in the Mammoth Cave are made without eyes. We never find an ear but where sound can put it in action; we never find a living thing, down to the invisible animalcule, that has not its appropriate nourishment at hand. And is it not strange that only a few of the thousands of diseases should have their appropriate remedies? Shall we call that "rational medicine" which teaches that sulphur will cure the itch, but denies that lime will cure a rash; believes that mercury will cure syphilis, but laughs at the idea of zinc as a remedy for herpes; knows that Peruvian bark will cure intermittent fever, but rejects the most positive testimony that belladonna will cure scarlet fever?

What can be the explanation of these inconsistencies? The professor furnishes a good answer — "It is so hard to get anything out of the dead hand of medical tradition."

Again: should that be called rational medicine of which its own chosen professor says, "The truth is, that medicine, professedly founded on observation, is as sensitive to outside influences, political, religious, philosophical, imaginative, as is the barometer to the changes of atmospheric density"? And this he proves by eight or ten pages of historic facts, showing the innumerable opinions and theories which have been set up, to be kicked over by the next man who should come along; — Dr. Rush charging Hippocrates with killing millions, by letting Nature loose upon sick people, and Sir John Forbes, Drs. Bigelow, Gould, Cotting, Hooker, and all other Hippocratic practitioners, holding Dr. Rush, and other heroic doctors, responsible for the lives of as many millions more. In the mean time all other branches of science have been steadily progressing — astronomy, chemistry, geology, constantly adding new principles and new facts, having no "counter currents," and never subject "to outside influences, political, religious, or imaginative."

Why is it that while all other branches of Science, including the collateral branches of Medicine, Anatomy, Physiology, Pathology, and Nosology, have so steadily advanced, Therapeutics, that important branch which regards the discovery and application of remedies for disease, has stood still for two thousand years?

The reason for this anomaly in science seems to be this: We have been fumbling at the door of Nature's great medical storehouse for six thousand years, in the dark, with the wrong key — one which never can unlock it.

Geology never did much while its "dead hand" held on to misinterpreted theology. Chemistry made no advances while it amused itself by chasing the phantoms of alchemy. Astronomy stood still till Galileo's telescope revealed the simple law which governs it. And Medical Science is drifted everywhere by "currents and counter currents," till it recognizes the simple law of Nature, which God, in infinite mercy, has given to guide it, — "*Similia similibus curantur.*" But wherever this law is recognized, the Science of Medicine has progressed as steadily as any other science.

Look at the Materia Medica of the two systems, as they have been developed by the last fifty years of time. Hundreds of articles have been tested by old school physicians on the sick, and thousands of patients have been killed in the experiments, as the doctors themselves acknowledge, and not a half dozen of all the medicines have continued in general use for any consecutive ten years of practice; while every article of well proved homeopathic medicine which was used fifty years ago is used now by every homeopathic physician. And of the hundreds of articles which have since been proved, by experiment (not on the sick, but on ourselves, thus avoiding the sacrifices consequent on old school experiments), not one that has been fairly proved to be useful is ever afterwards condemned or abandoned.

Experience (that is, experiment on the sick) can never open the treasures of medical science.

And yet this it is that has been "fostering chimerical hopes" since the world began.

The old school physicians, together with irregular practitioners, of all grades of intellect and acquirements, down to the meanest impostor that vends his well-known drugs under the guise of a new name, all trust to what they call experience; and this they have done from time immemorial. But experience, as a standard for testing the value of medicine, is not only fallacious, but is the basis of all empiricism, as we can readily show by a glance at its history.

Probably the first man or woman who felt a severe pain sought relief in some remedy. If relief came soon, that remedy had the credit of cure; if not, and other remedies were tried, the last experiment had the credit. Meantime Nature was making an effort to relieve the sufferer in her own way, and when relief came, who could tell whether it came on account of the medicine or in spite of it? If relief did not come, and the patient died, who could tell whether he died of the disease or the remedy?

Experiments, thus commenced, have been continued without any manifest improvement of system for six thousand years. Everything under heaven — animal, vegetable, mineral, or excrementitious — has been tried on some poor sick patient; thousands and even millions have been killed in these experiments, as the doctors themselves acknowledge; and every medicine in its turn has been condemned as injurious or useless, excepting six articles; and even these are not all fully admitted as specifics: Arsenic, Mercury, Sulphur, Cinchona, Iodine, and Colchicum. Here, then, we have the results of six thousand years of experiments with drugs on sick people; six medicines actually ascertained to be useful in as many different diseases — one for each millennium of experiment.

Besides these six articles of the *materia medica*, there is not one which is not discarded by many physicians as either injurious or useless, — some schools, and some neighborhoods of physicians, having confidence in one set of articles, and some in another, experimenting for a while with one article, and then leaving it for another.

Thus we have gone on, generation after generation, and century after century — everything else claiming to be scientific gradually improving; but old school therapeutics absolutely standing still: and these facts are freely admitted by our best physicians, as we have seen.

I remember being startled, forty years ago, while a

member of the Harvard School, by the announcement of the professor, then our oracle in Therapeutics, that after twenty-five years' experience in the use of emetics, as a means of breaking up fevers, he had just learned that his experience was useless. He supposed he had thus broken up hundreds of fevers; but by the experiments of the celebrated Louis of Paris, just then published, it had been proved that as many fevers would go on after an emetic as without one — thus proving worthless the experience in that matter of one of our most clear-headed and most observing professors. If such a man could not decide between the effects of medicine and the efforts of Nature, who could decide?

Louis also tested many other articles of the *materia medica*, and many other modes of treatment, with results equally humiliating to what is called experience in medicine. I give you a summary of statistics, collected from reliable authorities.

In cases of inflammation of the lungs, collected from hospitals in Glasgow, Vienna, London, Paris, and some other of the best hospitals in Europe, the percentage of death varied in direct proportion to the harshness of the treatment. Under the best old school physicians, it ranged from fourteen to twenty-four per cent., while the number of deaths of patients, with the same nursing, left to Nature, was only from seven to eight per cent. In this disease, therefore, medicine destroyed over seven per cent. of patients. In other diseases, where the treatment was less heroic, the percentage was less — four, and even three per cent.; but, on the other hand, in one hospital where bleeding and emetics were freely administered, more than twenty per cent. died — proving that two thirds of the deaths were produced by the treatment.

Surely these are not the legitimate effects of medicines, which are among the things pronounced by their Maker to be "very good." They are, however, the legitimate results of experiments on the sick, and are, it seems to me, sufficient to show that experience, as the means of developing medical resources, has proved a disastrous failure.

I have elsewhere shown that Nature is very lavish in her distributions of medical agents, furnishing them in the weeds, flowers, mineral combinations, and animal poisons; so that, everywhere, are found the means of alleviating sufferings and assisting Nature in the cure of disease. And is it reasonable that these inestimable blessings should be strewed in every pathway, and no means given to ascertain their healing virtues except by such miserable experiments on the sick as these to which we have referred? What might be expected, is found to be true, —

There is a simple law by which any medicine can be tested, and its virtues ascertained, with unerring certainty, without these dangerous experiments on the sick and suffering.

And the wonder is that for six thousand years the world should grope in darkness without discovering the light of it.

The naturalist will take a single bone of an animal

which he has never seen, and from it will construct the animal from which it was taken — show his disposition, the arrangements of his digestive organs, his habits, and the kind of food on which he was accustomed to live. All this is done by inductive reasoning, from the known uniformity of Nature's laws, as shown in the construction of different classes of animals.

The astronomer will watch the motion of a new comet, and, after a few nights or weeks, it may be, will tell you how far it is from the sun, how near it will ever go to it, how far off it will ever go, and when it will return. And this he does by induction from the laws which regulate the motion of heavenly bodies.

A careful observer will take a plant or a drug which he never before heard of, and, taking a portion of it himself, carefully watching its effects, and giving to twenty or thirty friends each equal portions, and noting the effects on each, will, with a few repetitions, get symptoms from which he can tell what disease, or combination of symptoms, that plant or drug is adapted to cure, with as perfect accuracy as the naturalist or the astronomer in the cases referred to. And his conclusions are formed by the same unerring process of induction from Nature's laws.

By this process have been tested, for the last fifty years and more, the virtues of very many medicines, every one of which, after millions of trials, is now used for the same symptoms of disease, and with the same satisfactory result as was obtained by them fifty years ago. Scientific physicians have since proved, in the same way, with more or less care, in all now over four hundred different medicines, every one of which that has been carefully proved to produce distinct symptoms on well persons, is confidently used to cure similar symptoms in the sick. And this is the simple law to which I referred.

Need I give you further evidence to prove the existence of a law by which to test the value of any medicine, without the miserable farce, or rather tragedy, of testing poisonous drugs on poor sick people? If further proof is needed of the truth and the value of this law, you have it in the results of its practice. Take, in the first place, diseases which appear in new forms, or rather, perhaps, in forms in which we are not accustomed to see them. We have not to hunt up precedents, or to wait to try experiments, but carefully noting the symptoms, and comparing them with the symptoms of different medicines, we select our remedy with almost unerring accuracy — at least with greater accuracy than, without this law, we could obtain by experience with the most familiar diseases. This advantage has been recently seen in diphtheria. Especially on its first advent to a city or neighborhood, the percentage of recovery has always been manifestly in favor of homeopathic treatment, where it has had a fair trial. But having no statistics to support this assertion, we can only appeal to general observations in regard to this disease.

But in cholera the advantage of homeopathy has been established beyond a question. In the aggregate of three thousand eight hundred and ninety-nine cases, in nine of the principal old school hospitals of Europe, there occurred two thousand and eighty-nine deaths — fifty-four per cent.; while in one thousand seven hundred and eighteen cases of the same epidemic, in six homeopathic hospitals, there occurred but five hundred and one deaths — twenty-nine per cent. — a mortality only about half as great. And in Edinburgh and Leith, as reported by the General Board of Health, in all the cases that occurred in four months, from October 4 to February 1, 1849, the deaths under old school practice were eighty-four and a half per cent., while under homeopathic treatment they were twenty-four and a half per cent. — three deaths to one. In some other diseases not new, the difference is less striking.

In pneumonia, in which we have seen that nearly one half the deaths were produced by crude drugs, one quarter were saved by homeopathic, compared with expectant. The exact statement is: —

Under homeopathic treatment, deaths 5 to 6 per cent.
Under allopathic treatment, deaths 14 to 24 per cent.
Under expectant,* deaths 7 to 8 per cent.

In typhus fever: —

Under homeopathic treatment, deaths $10\frac{6}{10}$ per cent.
Under allopathic treatment, deaths $21\frac{1}{10}$ per cent.
Under expectant, deaths $17\frac{5}{10}$ per cent.

* Trusting to Nature without medicines.

These statistics are from the Vienna hospitals, side by side for a period of three years, and show that in this disease four per cent. were lost by crude drugs, and seven per cent. were saved by homeopathic treatment, as compared with expectant, or do-nothing, treatment.

In diseases of children, as shown by statistics from the different orphan asylums in New York, the ratio of mortality, in a series of twelve years, was more than three to one in favor of homeopathic treatment, as seen by the medical report.

We have also the testimony of an old school physician, given under circumstances which make it significant and interesting. In 1852, Dr. Roath published in London a book which he entitled the "Fallacies of Homeopathy," which, he says, he was constrained to do, because "this system has unfortunately lately made, and continues to make, such progress in this country, and the metropolis in particular, and is daily extending its influence even amongst the most learned, and those whose high position in society gives them no little moral power over the opinions of the multitude, that our profession is, I think, bound to make it the subject of inquiry and investigation." To that end he collected statistics of different hospitals, to the number of thirty-two thousand six hundred and fifty-five homeopathic cases, and compared them with an equal number of cases from old school hospitals, honestly, I doubt not, intending to select cases so nearly alike as fairly to prove which was the best mode of treatment; but he was astonished to find that the mortality under old school treatment was $10\frac{5}{10}$ per cent., while under homeopathic treatment it was only $4\frac{4}{10}$ per cent. Still he was honest enough to publish the results; but, to let himself down gently, he thought the homeopathic cases must have been mild cases. His reasons for that opinion, however, I give in his own words: "Proportionally to their number of beds, they admit more patients, perhaps twice as many, as in other hospitals. And will not this be evidence that they have a large number of milder cases?" With this and two or three other similar efforts to nullify the influence of his own facts, he sends the book out to the London world to stop the influence of homeopathy amongst its "most learned citizens." How much influence it had among the citizens for whom it was intended, I have no means of knowing; but it certainly did help to establish the fact that homeopathy not only saves life, but cuts short diseases. What other reasonable explanation can be given to the fact that a greater number, by nearly one half, was admitted to the same beds, than that by the same proportion the diseases were cut shorter? And this inference is corroborated by other statistics, as follows:—

By statistics from the same source as that of those before given, it is shown that the mean duration of pneumonia was,—

Under homeopathic treatment, $11\frac{2}{3}$ days.
Under old school treatment, 29 days.
Under do-nothing treatment, 20 days.

Showing, that while it takes longer to get well by old school treatment than by trusting to Nature, it takes much less than half the time to get well of pneumonia under homeopathic treatment.

Dr. Kurtz compiled a table of the mean duration of all diseases in the hospitals of Paris, Berlin, and Gottingen, under old school treatment, as compared with the hospitals of Vienna, Munich, and Leipzig, under homeopathic treatment; and the average was, —

Under old school, 28 days.
Under homeopathic, 20 days.

A saving of more than one quarter of the time. These statistics show the error of our enemies, who insist that "Homeopathy is a specious mode of doing nothing" — proving as they do, incontestably, that in the gravest diseases it both saves life and cuts short disease. And this accords with the testimony of all who have compared it, as many of us have, with the expectant as well as with the heroic mode of treatment. But do not the imagination, change of diet and regimen, often have an effect which is mistaken for the effect of medicine? Undoubtedly, in some cases; but in other cases the proof is irresistible that no such influences exist.

Take, besides the statistics already given, chronic cases of disease, especially of children, which are treated without change of diet or regimen, and such explanations are, of course, inadmissible. Scores of such cases can be collected from the books of homeopathic physicians in Boston, who would testify that they have seen the effects of homeopathic medicine under circumstances which preclude the idea that Nature, or change of diet, or regimen, or imagination, can come in to deceive them. Of hundreds of such cases take one: —

A child, three years old, had been wasting away with diarrhœa, vomiting of food, and restlessness, pain and sleeplessness, for eighteen months. Advice from various sources had been taken; but getting discouraged, for six months nothing had been done but to feed it with milk, of which it could bear but very little.

It was a mere skeleton, with a wrinkled skin hanging loosely upon it. Its parents, supposing it was soon to die, asked for homeopathic medicine to help it to die comfortably. One globule of arsenic was given at night, so diluted that a dose could be given to every man, woman, and child in Massachusetts without consuming a single grain; and, for the first time for months, that night it slept well, without vomiting its milk.

No change was made in any of its circumstances, and no medicine was given except one such globule every second night; and in two months it had gained flesh, and was well. If this case were solitary, it might be considered a wonderful coincidence; but similar cases, occurring almost daily, afford conclusive evidence of the power of homeopathic medicine in doses at first sight ridiculously inadequate to the effects claimed for them. But analogous facts in Nature are seen all about us, which ought to show the absurdity of refusing to investigate homeopathy on account of its claims to infinitesimal influences.

A man dies in awful agony, after indescribable suffering, because a particle of saliva from a rabid dog has entered the skin by, perhaps, a very slight scratch. The amount of poison that produced these terrible effects may have been so perfectly infinitesimal that no chemical or other test could detect a difference between the saliva which produced that effect and the saliva of a healthy dog.

Again: the microscope can scarcely detect, and the senses cannot recognize, the infinitesimal particles of malaria which, conveyed in the atmosphere, and taken into the human system, produce chills and fever, and internal derangements that last for years, and often produce death.

Cases are also known of individuals so susceptible to an influence from dry ipecac that they are thrown into frightful spasms and such stridulous breathing as to endanger life in some cases, even in the room adjoining that in which it is being put up in a small quantity. Many a man, also, has had his eyes shut up, and been kept at home for days and weeks, because he went into the neighborhood of ivy or dogwood.

Cases, too, of severe inflammation and fever have been produced by aroma from roses, almost realizing the poetic idea of "dying of a rose, in aromatic pain;" and other instances of infinitesimal influence on the human system in health will occur to the mind of every careful observer. And shall we refuse to admit the possibility of similar influences on the more susceptible human system when diseased?

Indeed, it is admitted by all old school physicians that the articles of medicine called specifics will produce an effect in very small doses. Fowler's Solution is a form of arsenic more used than any other, in doses as small as those given by many homeopathic physicians.

Many other of the empirical preparations which have been analyzed and adopted by the faculty, owe their virtues to exceedingly minute portions of corrosive sublimate or other medicines. Iodine inhalations also are but the homeopathic use of that drug, for we find it makes no difference how a medicine is introduced into the system, whether by inhalation, absorption, or through the mouth and stomach. But the most marvellous example of the practice of homeopathy, without knowing it, is seen in what is called subcutaneous injections, where very small quantities of medicine are inserted under the skin with wonderful effect. Dr. James McCrath, of the British Seamen's Hospital in Smyrna, published in Braithwaite's Journal a report of fifty cases of intermittent fever treated by one or two grains of quinine injected into the skin of the arm, and the results were more satisfactory than in patients treated by twenty grains by the mouth; and he says that Dr. Chesseaud (who introduced it) will have a right to a reward from all civilized governments in the world, seeing the immense economy of quinine it will effect in all hospitals. Now, it is easy to bring a thousand cases of cure of intermittent fever by homeopathic doses of quinine vastly less than those injected into the arm; but we have never thought of getting a patent on account of the economy of the practice. Sulphur and iodine are also acknowledged to do good in springs but very slightly impregnated with them; and thus we have an acknowledgment that all the specifics can produce their effect in very small doses. See, too, the reasonableness of the homeopathic idea that the specific influence of drugs is not dependent on the quantity or strength of the medicine used, all that is useful in a medicine being as well obtained from a little as from more.

Hydrophobia is just as fatal when induced by the slightest scratch from the poisoned tooth as when produced by severe laceration. Intermittent fever is as severe when induced by a single hour of exposure to its malaria as when under its influence for months. Poison from ivy or dogwood is just as severe if induced by passing near it as by handling or chewing it. Vaccination is as effectual when induced by matter from the point of a needle as the point of a jackknife, and small-pox is no more likely to be fatal when taken from one dying with the disease than when taken from the mildest case of varioloid.

The specific influence, in these cases, may be more sure to follow a thorough than a slight inoculation; but if any effect at all is produced, it seems to be the same in either case.

Analogous to these effects seem to be the specific effects of homeopathic medicine; so that while nothing can be more clearly proved than the homeopathic law that medicines which in large doses will produce symptoms of disease will in small doses cure similar symptoms, yet it may be difficult to decide whether the tenth or the ten-thousandth of a grain is the best dose. Indeed, the limit beyond which a medicine can be so attenuated as to cease to produce its specific effect has never been ascertained. But, practically, it is only important to ascertain what dose is most sure to do good without the power of doing harm.

For example: the tenth of a grain of nux vomica will cure a certain form of sick headache, and it is claimed that the trillionth of a grain will do the same thing; but it is possible that the tenth may be capable of doing some harm by inducing other symptoms of disease, while, on the other hand, the high dilution, being more influenced by surrounding circumstances, may be more uncertain, while a medium attenuation might avoid either evil. The one dose is as truly homeopathic as the other, and, by analogy with other influences just cited, one dose may produce equal effects with the other. While, therefore, we may see no advantage in adopting high dilutions, we should, at least, be taught, by analogous influences, not to ridicule them.

While visiting a patient, on the day of the annular eclipse in 1830, I found a man in bed in the middle of the forenoon. I asked him if he was sick. He said No, but he had heard there was to be a terrible eclipse, and he staid in bed. I asked his views of astronomy, but he said he knew nothing about astronomy, and he wouldn't know anything about it, the thing was so absurd. "Why," said he, "how could I lie in bed with the world t'other side up half of the time?" The argument was certainly plausible, but it neither convinced astronomers of error in their calculations, nor did it stop the eclipse. The idea of the absurdity of the rotation of the earth so blinded him, that he did not see that he was doing homage to astronomy by his very fears of an eclipse according to astronomical calculation.

Not exactly a parallel is seen in those who will not investigate the principles of homeopathy because of the absurdity of the idea of power in infinitesimal doses. But I have lately met a case more nearly parallel, in a doctor who would not investigate the infinitesimal humbug, or any other humbug, but who has made a patient believe that a lameness of the knees was caused by homeopathic medicine settling in them. The patient had taken, perhaps, the millionth of a grain of medicine, every night, for some weeks. The doctor had seen a number of cases before where homeopathic medicine had produced a similar effect.

But how decide, when doctors disagree? Why not put us on our reasons and our facts, and decide from them? Suppose the question before us was, Which is safest and most comfortable for a passage across the Atlantic, a wind-ship or a steamship? An experienced ship-master tells you the wind-ship is safest and best; he has tried them for years, and he knows; he would on no account trust himself in a steamship; it might blow up. But another master, who has tried both, says the steamship is safest and most comfortable; and he tells you why, and offers statistics to prove his position. Whose testimony will you take? We offer the testimony of those who have tried both modes of practice, that homeopathy is a fixed law of Nature; that it is the safest, quickest, and most reliable mode of cure in the gravest diseases; and we offer to show you that its principles are in harmony with all of Nature's laws, and therefore reasonable. Let us, for a moment, compare the deductions from this law with the teachings of old school therapeutics, and see which is most reasonable.

It is admitted that six medicines are capable of curing six different forms of disease. Is it reasonable that all other medicines should be so constituted as to do more harm than good? Sulphur will cure the itch, mercury will cure syphilis, quinine will cure fever and ague, iodine will cure goitre, colchicum will cure some forms of rheumatism, and arsenic will cure a disease of the skin. But according to old school doctrines, all other diseases are safest in the hands of Nature, or at least have no medicine specifically provided for them, while all other medicines, doing more harm than good, might, but for the welfare of the fishes, be sunk in the bottom of the sea.

There are known to be thousands of medicines as capable of affecting the human system as arsenic, or mercury, or quinine, or sulphur, or iodine, or colchicum; and thousands of diseases as distinct in their manifestations as those which are cured by these medicines. And yet, according to old school theory, these six articles are all that are adapted to cure any particular form of disease. Does this accord with the uniformity of Nature's common laws? Now compare this theory with deductions from the homeopathic law, and see which is most reasonable. It is admitted that six medicines, by a secret power, to use the words of Dr. Bigelow, "produce a change in the system favorable to recovery from disease," and that in doses so small as to be tasteless and to produce no injury.

From this fact we infer that all other medicines were intended to act in the same way on their own appropriate diseases, and this inference is corroborated, and proved beyond reasonable controversy, by the homeopathic proof that at least four hundred other medicines do produce similar effects on as many different forms of disease. Will any man, claiming to understand Nature's laws, say that this homeopathic inference is unreasonable?

The susceptibility of drugs to do evil is evidently given them to show us what diseases they are capable of curing; and by rightly using these evils we convert them into blessings. Every case of poisoning from arsenic, mercury, belladonna, aconite, or any other drug that was ever recorded, is made the means of relieving similar suffering by the use of the same medicines in homeopathic practice. The only use homeopathists make of crude drugs is to study their evil influences, and use the same remedies in homeopathic doses to relieve similar symptoms of disease: this we do every day. Can we believe that our heavenly Father intends that, when suffering from pain and sickness, we should add to our suffering by taking disgusting drugs which are in themselves evils, and that we should make no effort to make them palatable and innoxious? Our food is furnished us in a crude, unpalatable condition; but we have intellects to adapt it to our taste and requirements, and when we rightly use them, we both relish it and are conscious of its adaptation to our wants. So God evidently intended we should use our reason in adapting crude medicines to our taste and requirements, and when we do so, we are rewarded by the same evidence of its adaptation. If, instead of relief, we get evils from medicine, we may be sure we have mistaken the remedy or have given it in an improper condition or quantity, just as we are always sure we have taken improper food, if, instead of gratified appetite, we get disturbance from it. Other animals are furnished both with food and medicine in a state adapted to their wants, because they have not sense to prepare them. The sick cat takes with relish the simple catnip provided for it, and suffers no evils from it; but the sick child must swallow drugs which it shudders to think of, and which disturbs all its functions for days and weeks, and sometimes for life. Surely it is reasonable to suppose our children are to be as kindly cared for when sick as our cats. Would our kind heavenly Father so carefully provide for us in health as to give us enjoyment in the use of everything adapted to our wants, and when sick consign us to blisters, hot irons, cataplasms, and disgusting drugs? Our reason, therefore, as well as our humanity and our experience, accords with the fair deductions from the homeopathic law, and demands that all things "in themselves evils," or offensive to the patient, whether of diet, regimen, or medicine, should be excluded from the sick chamber or hospital.

These facts and deductions seem to me to be true and sound. If they are false or defective, no one need be deceived by them. If they are right, the following conclusions are irresistible: —

1st. That in Physiology, Pathology, Nosology, and everything pertaining to the management of patients, except Therapeutics, the old school and the homeopathic agree.

2d. That in Therapeutics, old school practitioners have no standard but experience, and no means of testing the value of medicine but experiments on the sick, which they have in common with all classes of empirics, and which they acknowledge to have been the means of killing millions of patients.

3d. That the result of all this sacrifice, and the experience of six thousand years, has only established the fact that six medicines are useful in as many different diseases, and that all other articles of the *materia medica*, as now used, are either useless, or do more harm than good; but that, nevertheless, these dangerous experiments are still being tried, some doctors having faith in one article and some in another.

4th. That homeopathists have discovered a law of Nature by which, without experimenting on the sick, the virtues of all medicines can be tested, and the symptoms of disease ascertained, which each is adapted to cure.

5th. That, by the application of this law, over three hundred medicines have already been proved, and have the confidence of all homeopathic practitioners, some fifty of which have been used for more than fifty years for the same symptoms of disease, and with the same satisfactory results; and that doctors who have practised both ways declare that many diseases considered incurable by old school treatment are proved to be curable by homeopathic treatment.

6th. That it is susceptible of proof, that under the same collateral circumstances, homeopathic will save fifty per cent. more of life than old school treatment.

7th. That it saves all the suffering from lancets, hot irons, caustics, cataplasms, emetics, cathartics, and the whole paraphernalia of torments which so terrify patients, and so disgrace the profession, to say nothing of drug diseases, which are entailed on almost all who take poisonous medicines in large doses; saves at least one quarter of the time of the patient, and consequently one quarter of his average expense of treatment, besides saving at least nine tenths of the expense of medicines; and this last item is not inconsiderable, the Apothecary's Report for Bellevue Hospital for 1856 showing a disbursement of nearly five thousand dollars for drugs and medicines.

8th. That its doctrines and practices are all consonant with Nature's common laws, and all commend themselves to the common sense of all intelligent men who understand and practise them.

The only difference between us and the Nature-trusting practitioners of Boston is this: they believe that Nature will generally cure acute diseases, and the doctor's duty consists in protecting the patient from harmful influences, directing the diet and regimen, and inspiring the confidence of both patient and friends. All this we do, and give besides, in all cases, medicines which never interfere with Nature's efforts, but, if rightly selected, assist her, and hasten the process of cure. How much more do old school practitioners differ among themselves! One class thinks, with Sir Astley Cooper, that "medication does more harm than good," and therefore practise as I have intimated, leaving almost all diseases to Nature; while another class thinks, with Dr. Rush, that "millions have been killed by letting Nature loose on sick people," and therefore take almost all diseases out of Nature's hands. One thinks opium and alcohol are the two most valuable articles of the *materia medica*. Another believes that no two articles have done, and are now doing, so much mischief in the world.

Chemical laws are no more certain in their operation than is the homeopathic law, and this I assert after twenty consecutive years of practice in experimental chemistry. I am no more sure that an appropriate quantity of acid will neutralize a given quantity of alkali than I am sure that a medicine which in large doses will produce a headache, will in small doses cure a similar headache. Chemistry, therefore, to my mind, is no more entitled to be ranked as a science than is homeopathy.

Thousands of educated physicians have tested it in practice; but not one, to my knowledge, ever found a fact or an argument to disprove, or, after the trial of a single year, ever disbelieved it. Indeed, the idea of turning back again to what is technically called Rational Medicine is as preposterous as the idea of turning a disciple of Galileo to a belief in the old Ptolemaic system of astronomy.

Ridicule of Homeopathy.

Some sage contemporary might say to Galileo, I don't believe in your philosophy, for the world could not turn round without spilling the water from my well; but Galileo would reply, as he did, "Nevertheless, the world does turn round, and I can prove it." So some equally sage professor may say, I don't believe in homeopathy, for I have never seen much effect on the waters of Lake Superior by a drowned louse;* nevertheless, the law, "*Similia similibus curantur*," is true, and we can prove it; and this is all we claim for homeopathy. The Professor says, "Hahnemann believed in infinitesimal doses, and in psora as the origin of many chronic diseases; and does not Hahnemann himself represent homeopathy as it now exists?" "He certainly ought to be its best representative," &c.

Admit that Hahnemann, in his dotage, did believe and publish some foolish things; is homeopathy respon-

* See "Currents and Counter Currents in Medical Science," by Professor O. W. Holmes.

sible for them, even while they were never adopted as the homeopathic creed? And is Rational Medicine responsible for every foolish thing its professors believe and publish? Let us try on a case, and see how it fits. I cannot believe, with the rationalist, that typhoid fever resides on the mucous membrane of the tongue, and can be scraped off with a hoe. And does any rational practitioner say, Neither do I believe such nonsense; but "does not" your own Professor of your own favorite school "represent" rational medicine "as it now exists"? "He certainly ought to be its best representative." And does he not, in this very address, recommend a hoe as a very economical remedy — "better than many a prescription with a split-footed ℞ before it"? And does he not enforce his recommendation by a very interesting scrap of colonial history, the pith of which is that Winslow scraped the tongue of Massasoit, then like to die of typhoid fever, and thus saved his life, and with it the colony?

Here is proof that the Professor believes that typhoid fever resides on the tongue, for how else could it be scraped off. And thus we establish the very important discovery in rational medicine: typhoid fever is a disease of the tongue, and a hoe will cure it.

Now, ridiculous as is this representation of rational medicine, it is less a caricature than any published representation of homeopathic doctrines which I can find from the pen of any old school practitioner within the last thirty years. See the Professor's representation of us in this very address.

After charging us with "outraging human nature with infusions of *pediculus capitis*, — that is, of course, as we understand their dilutions, the names of these things; for if a fine-tooth-comb insect were drowned in Lake Superior, we cannot agree with them in thinking that every drop of its waters would be impregnated with all the pedicular virtues they so highly value," — he says: "They know what they are doing — they are appealing to the detestable old superstitious presumption in favor of whatever is nauseous and noxious as being good for the sick." Here are three distinct misrepresentations of us in one sentence: —

1. We are represented as "outraging human nature," and appealing to the vulgar and "superstitious presumption in favor of whatever is nauseous," and this under a Latin name, and "in infinitesimal sugar globules," while, in the very preceding paragraph, he has been referring to the allopathic use of medicines, "transcendently unmentionable," and of "unlovely secretions," which were used undiluted.

2. We are represented as believing that a louse, drowned in any part of Lake Superior, would impregnate its waters a hundred miles off, against all "currents and counter currents" — a belief which no one "outside of the walls of Bedlam" ever entertained.

3. We are represented as highly valuing the virtues of the *pediculus capitis*, when it cannot be found in any list of homeopathic remedies, and, I venture the assertion, was never used by a respectable homeopathic physician in any dilution. As a homeopathic remedy,

it seems to have come from the *head* of his friend, Dr. Martin, who charges us with hooking the louse from the allopathic *materia medica*, with fifty other articles, some of which are among our most valuable remedies. This one, however, he acknowledges he cannot find in our list of remedies, or anywhere else; but he *understands* "it enjoys a distinguished place in homeopathic pharmacy." *

This address, by the way, affords another illustration of the usual method of attack on homeopathy — by misrepresentation, rather than by facts or arguments. The main purpose seems to be to show that homeopathy did not originate with Hahnemann. And this he attempts to do by hunting up all the medicines from the animal, vegetable, or mineral kingdoms used by Hahnemann, and then going back hundreds of years to see how many of the same medicines had been used before Hahnemann was born. But as he finds among old school medicines *everything under heaven*, he has left poor Hahnemann no other resources but their *materia medica*. And what does he prove by that process?

But what seems most to amuse the doctor is, that he finds Hahnemann guilty of hooking from their *materia medica* inert substances, as gold, antimony, tin, silica, &c., and pretending to perform wonderful cures with them, after trituration with sugar. But does he forget that lead and mercury are equally inert substances? What is his blue pill, which has cured so many and

* See Address of Henry A. Martin, M. D., of Roxbury, before the Norfolk County Medical Society, page 26.

killed so many patients, but crude mercury — of which a pound could be taken with impunity — and conserve of roses, perseveringly triturated together? Apropos to our triturations, which are sources of such infinite amusement, let us remind him of the well-known fact that old school doctors attribute the power of the blue pill to such a minute division of the mercurial particles as to adapt them to the capacity of the absorbent vessels. Whether their theory be right or not, every homeopathic physician knows that gold, and charcoal, and silica, and many other inert substances, are made active and valuable medicines by a similar process, using only sugar, instead of conserve of roses, as a medium by which to unite them with oxygen.

The address closes with deep regrets that he had so exhausted the time in these, to him, very interesting researches that he could not, as he intended, bring out his plan for punishing such incorrigible quacks. But whether it was his design to punish them for hooking his *pediculus capitis*, or for copying his *placebo* practice, he does not inform us. One or the other it must be, for neither he nor his contemporaries charge us with any worse sins.

Misrepresentation of Homeopathy.

Neither does the original exponent of Rational Medicine in New England ever refer to homeopathy, to my knowledge, without misrepresenting it. In his last work on Rational Medicine he even charges us with being faithless to our principles.* He says: "There is great reason to believe that homeopathic faith is not always kept up to its original purity by its professors; traces of the occasional use of very heroic medicines are often detected," &c.

Will the doctor be kind enough to refer to any article of homeopathic faith that specifies the size or strength of the dose at all. The only rule is to give enough to produce the effect desired. And now that the doctor is up, let me relieve his mind on another point. He says, on the same page, "The man must be somewhat of a stoic who can look upon a case of severe colic, and quiet his conscience with administering inappreciable globules, instead of remedies." Now, let me tell my kind-hearted old friend and teacher, what I know to be true, after repeated experiments, both in accordance with the rules of Bigelow's Sequel and those of homeopathy, that a homeopathic remedy will relieve the severest colic in one quarter of the time of his own most heroic opiate; often before it could be obtained from the nearest druggist. Opium is the slow coach, for which we are not willing to wait.

But is not the dose which homeopathic practitioners generally give so ridiculously small as to justify the definition given to our system, by expositors of Rational Medicine, "as a specious mode of doing nothing"? To one accustomed to the use of ipecac, for example, in twenty grain doses, it may seem impossible that the

* Expositions of Rational Medicine. By Jacob Bigelow, M. D.

one thousandth part of a grain of the same article can produce any effect. But how is it known that twenty grains produce an emetic effect, but by experiment? And experiment as clearly shows that the one thousandth part of a grain of ipecac will as surely stop vomiting, when produced by some other cause. And how can the Professor know, or any one else, whether the ten thousandth part of a grain might not also produce an effect? Theoretically, who shall decide whether the crude article, third, or thirtieth dilution, is best adapted to the capacity and size of the invisible capillaries in which it must circulate and on which it must act, or whether one dilution may not be best adapted to diseases of one tissue, and another to diseases of a different tissue?

We can easily ridicule the high dilutions, but who shall settle that old question of divisibility, so as to tell us in which dilution, from the third to thirtieth, the original material has ceased to exist, or existing, is too fine to be adapted to the infinitesimal vessels of which the tissues are composed?

Take, for example, sulphate of copper, one grain of which can be seen intermingled with every drop of five gallons of water, which may be equal to the fifth dilution. Does it cease to exist in the sixth dilution, because it cannot be seen?

Old School Physicians prescribe on Homeopathic Principles without knowing it.

Who knows the nature of the specific action of medicines, whether it may not be increased by the increase of surface produced by each dilution, just as the power of electricity may be increased by extending the surface? The action of medicine is a mystery always; and is it profitable to ridicule that of which we know nothing?

And how do the specifics act in the cure of disease? All classes of practitioners have seen the hundredth part of a grain of corrosive sublimate, given in repeated doses, gradually change a diseased action to a healthy action. Call this an alterative, or call it a homeopathic action. What is it? In Bigelow's Sequel you are told, "Alterative is a name applied to substances which are found to produce a change in the system favorable to the recovery from disease." And he gives, as examples, arsenic, sulphur, mercury. The same articles, it will be remembered, which are mentioned by our Professor as the specifics; and these articles are found to produce their effect in very small doses.

Here is homeopathy on a small scale. Three or four hundred articles besides those mentioned by the Professor and the Doctor, are also known to homeopathic practitioners to "produce a change in the system favorable to recovery from disease," and their number is constantly increasing, and the fair inference is, that all other medical substances are intended to act in the same way on their own appropriate diseases.

But *old school practitioners and Rational professors can see no common sense in homeopathy.*

Will the Professor's six methods of "misapplying the evidence of Nature," give us a clew to the reason of this anomaly? Let us see. He says, — *

First. "There is the natural incapacity for sound observation." "We see this in many persons who know a *good deal about books*, but who are not sharp-sighted enough to buy a horse or deal with human diseases." A truth that cannot be better illustrated than by reference to the treatment of typhoid fever with a hoe.

Secondly. "There is, in some persons, a singular inability to weigh the value of testimony, of which, I think, from a pretty careful examination of his books, Hahnemann affords the best specimen outside of the walls of Bedlam." That Hahnemann is the best specimen outside of Bedlam, we certainly cannot agree, for we have seen a Professor who believes, from mere tradition, that a hoe will cure typhoid fever, but ridicules the testimony of hundreds of educated physicians, that belladonna will cure a sore throat, and aconite a fever.

Thirdly. "We are led into inveterate logical errors, by counting only favorable cases." And here the Professor supplies an illustration. If an Indian chief gets well of typhoid fever after hoeing out his mouth, his case is reported; but nothing is said of the other poor Indians who died in spite of the scraping.

Fourthly. "The *post hoc ergo propter hoc* error." "That is, he got well after taking medicine, therefore,

* Currents and Counter Currents in Medical Science.

in consequence of taking it." Let us look again to the same source for illustration. Massasoit got well after scraping his tongue, therefore the hoe saved his life, "and saved the colony, and thus rendered Massachusetts and the Massachusetts Medical Society a possibility." "*Post hoc ergo propter hoc.*"

Lastly. "A reason for the golden tooth,"—"that is, assuming a falsehood for a fact, and giving reasons for it." This the Professor illustrates by the "homeopathic materia medica." But the homeopathic materia medica is founded on proof, and nothing but proof admits a single article, as has been explained. But what well-attested fact is his own hoe theory founded on? Indeed, every practical physician knows the statement "that the condition of the tongue does not in the least imply that of the stomach" to be untrue.

Who practises Deception in Medicine?

But suppose our system is "a specious mode of doing nothing," and our "Materia Medica sugar of milk and a nomenclature," are we sinners above all others? By their own showing we carry out the plan of Hippocrates, and Bigelow, and Cotting, and the Professor himself; for we certainly give Nature a fair chance, and our "rules of diet and nursing are excellent," Miss Nightingale being judge (and her authority will, of course, be accepted by the Professor, who places her name next to that of Hippocrates). What, then, is the offence for which we are treated with such contempt by our allopathic brethren? Why, we give sugar of milk, and make our patients think we are doing something for them. That we use the slightest deception, is not true; but, if it were, are we the only practitioners who deceive patients with "sugar of milk and a nomenclature"?

Look at the piles of prescriptions put up every day by every apothecary in Boston, and remember, that according to the Professor, you are at the American headquarters of the "Nature-trusting" practice. How many of them contain anything more important than sugar of milk, with, perhaps, a little coloring matter? And remember that every prescription costs the patient from twenty-five to fifty cents, while our medicine costs the patient nothing; and then ask Dr. Howe's least promising pupil whether the homeopathic or the rational practitioner is most amenable to the charge of deceiving with placebo medicines. And that is all the charge that our worst enemies bring against us. By this comparison, it will be seen that I have presented the worst view of homeopathy, and the best view of old practice.

For while it is evident, as I have shown, that one class of practitioners is every day practising deception, by writing placebo prescriptions, to be paid for, in which they have not themselves the slightest confidence (the only object being to please the patient, while Nature cures the disease), another class is doing infinitely worse — writing for medicines, to be paid for, which actually do very great harm. That too much medicine is given, the Professor proves by reference to the undisputed fact, that doctors and their families take little or no medicine, and, for the inference from this fact, he appeals to "the least promising of Dr. Howe's pupils."

And here, by the way, I wish to present to the same sapient umpire a counter statement, equally true. Homeopathic physicians and their families do take their own medicine, and in precisely the same doses and dilutions as their other patients take them. Apropos to the charge of deception, I will state a bit of experience.

For twenty years, up to 1845, I studied and practised medicine in the confidence of the Massachusetts Medical Society; but, like most of my fellows, I gradually lost confidence in medicine, till my practice was as harmless as the most perfect "Nature-trusting" practitioner of Boston or vicinity; but my conscience gave me so much trouble while practising the deception, absolutely necessary in order to retain my patients till Nature cured the disease, that I wrote my last placebo prescription in 1845, resolving that, come what would, I would live in peace with conscience. Having thus cast off the fear of the Medical Society, I was enabled to look at facts, all about me, showing the truth and the success of homeopathy, and the result was an honest adoption of its principles and its practice.

And now, having no occasion for deception in order to retain my patients, and giving no medicine but with the honest purpose and expectation of curing disease, or at least of assisting Nature in doing so, and receiving almost daily acknowledgments of cure, where Nature and heroic remedies have all failed, I enjoy the practice of medicine as I did not think it possible while in old school practice. True, it is not pleasant to see such epithets as "Arrant Quackery," "Infinitesimal Humbug," "Solemn Farce," "Pretended Science," &c., applied to that system, which, next to the *Christian religion*, we esteem the best gift of God to man; but when we see, as in the Professor's address,* these opprobrious terms applied to us in six different places, without one fact or argument to show their application, we believe, as everybody else believes, that facts and arguments would not be withheld, but for the want of them. And when these very men, who send every day prescriptions, to be paid for, which they know to be worthless, refuse to consult with us in cases of surgery or obstetrics, where we should not differ in practice, making no other charge against us than that we give "sugar of milk," we can heartily join, with our intelligent neighbors, in the laugh at their ridiculous position, especially as they who *win* are always allowed to laugh.

Professional Courtesy.

A case of the latter kind occurred in my own practice, sufficiently instructive, not to say amusing, to warrant a brief narration. A lady in one of our best families, a favorite in a large circle of friends, was in a

* Currents and Counter Currents in Medical Science.

condition almost desperate; and wanting advice and assistance, I recommended a friend of great experience in such cases; but in the consternation of the neighborhood, and in the absence of the husband, each kind-hearted neighbor proposed sending for *her* doctor, as all would then be safe. One ran for an old allopathic friend of the family; but he absolutely refused to go to the house, even to save the life of a daughter of an old friend.

Another was hastily sent for, who happened to be my junior in the Harvard School, and my junior in the Medical Society, Dean of the Faculty, Professor of Obstetrics, &c., &c. He *would go*, as an act of humanity, but with the distinct understanding that he did not consult with a homeopathic physician. He did go, and walking, with solemn tread, into the chamber, he "whipped the devil around the stump," by looking straight at the bed-post, at which I was standing, and consulting *that*, and giving to *that* his advice; thus ingeniously evading the medical law, but, apparently, not quite satisfying his own conscience, for he went out of the house as if the very —— Medical Society were at his heels, kindly hinting that he should be willing to call again, and do what could be done for the suffering patient, provided the homeopathic doctor could be disposed of.

The father, himself not a believer in homeopathy, indignant at the "solemn farce," said to me, "I can stand no more of this nonsense; do what you think best, get what assistance you choose, and I will take the responsibility;" shrewdly inquiring if these doctors had not lost patients by homeopathy. And his intimation that the Medical Society was not fully responsible for all he had seen and heard, was corroborated by the fact, that another friend of the family, a physician of high standing, had heard of no law against consulting with an educated physician, if he did give sugar pills instead of placebo prescriptions. The result was, a free and gentlemanly attendance and assistance, till, by the blessing of God on a course of treatment quite different from that recommended through the bed-post, our patient recovered.

THE CRUSADE AGAINST HOMEOPATHY.

HERE let us leave "The Currents and Counter Currents in Medical Science," and, borrowing the motto of another celebrated author, close this part of the subject by recounting, very briefly, "The Happy Success of the Valiant Knight, and his Dreadful and Inconceivable Adventures; with other Incidents worthy to be recorded by the most able Historian."

The crusade against homeopathy in New England was commenced in 1841 by the same Professor whom we have before quoted, and was announced in these words: "I shall treat it, not by ridicule, but by argument;" "with a firm belief that its pretensions and assertions cannot stand before a single hour of calm investigation." *

The address is commenced with the acknowledgment that "The one great doctrine which constitutes the basis of homeopathy, as a system, is expressed by the Latin aphorism, *Similia similibus curantur.*" And yet, without bringing a single argument against this one great doctrine, he devotes the rest of his lecture to a mere effigy, which he makes up of rags and shreds from the mind of Hahnemann in his dotage, which he labels homeopathy; but which is as unlike it as Don Quixote's

* Homeopathy and its Kindred Delusions, page 27.

windmills were unlike the giants for which he mistook them.

In a Western village, in 1860, when Republicanism was carrying all before it, according to the papers, some sapient politicians adopted a new and safe way of combatting it. They obtained some old clothes, stuffed them with straw, and labelling their effigy "Old Abe," danced around it like the Professor's typhoid Indians, "making such a hellish noise as they probably thought would scare away the devil of" * Republicanism. They finally pelted it with stones, and, demolishing it, seemed to think they had put an end to Republicanism. So our hero, having in less than an hour demolished his own effigy of Hahnemann, seemed to think he had kept his engagement, and demolished homeopathy past resuscitation; indeed, he was so sure of its death that he gravely proceeded to *post mortem* arrangements. This part of the service is sufficiently amusing to warrant a copy of the programme verbatim, with a few running commentaries.

The Professor says: "It only remains to throw out a few conjectures as to *the particular manner* in which it is to break up and disappear."

"1. The confidence of the few believers in this delusion will never survive the loss of friends, who may die of any acute disease, under a treatment such as that prescribed by homeopathy. It is doubtful how far cases of this kind will be trusted to its mercies; but,

* Address of O. W. Holmes, M. D., May 30, 1860, page 23.

wherever it acquires any considerable foothold, such cases must come, and with them the ruin of those who practise it, should any highly valuable life be thus sacrificed."

Well, twenty-seven years have passed away since this terrible doom was assigned us, and "we still live."

"2. After its novelty has worn out, the ardent and capricious individuals who constitute the most prominent class of its patrons will return to visible doses, were it only for the sake of a change."

As a commentary on this prophecy, I simply challenge contradiction to the following statement: For every family that gives up homeopathic for the old school practice, fifty give up old school for homeopathic practice.

"3. The semi-homeopathic practitioner will gradually withdraw from the *rotten half* of his business, and try to make the public forget his connection with it."

This prophecy has proved literally true; but not exactly in the manner intended by the prophet. Every man of us who began practising both ways (and nine tenths of us began that way), finding, by experience, that homeopathic practice is the most reliable, safe, and expeditious mode of curing disease, have gradually withdrawn from allopathy, till, after a very few years, we give up "*the rotten half*" altogether. To this there is not a known exception.

"4. The ultra homeopathist will either recant and try to rejoin the medical profession, or he will embrace some newer, and, if possible, equally extravagant doctrine, or he will stick to his colors, and go down with his sinking doctrine. *Very few will pursue the course last mentioned.*"

When this prediction was published, there were probably in Massachusetts seven or eight educated homeopathic physicians, now there are about three hundred; then there were in the United States probably one hundred, now probably at least four thousand; then the prophet had just reported homeopathy in Paris to be in a "condition sufficiently miserable," — to use his own words, — and going down, as it was also, according to the same authority, in England and Germany; now there are in Paris probably two hundred educated homeopathic practitioners; and in every place where homeopathy has obtained a foothold it has steadily progressed. Not a man of all this army of homeopathic physicians has ever been known to recant, and not one has embraced any newer doctrine, extravagant or otherwise, except as an adjuvant to homeopathy.

Of its present condition you can judge by the following facts: Of the principal royal families in Europe a large majority are under the care of homeopathic physicians; — that of the Emperor of France, and the Emperor of Russia, and of the Kings of Italy, Prussia, Belgium, Hanover, Bavaria, and Netherlands, and the Queen of Spain, as well as many of the Austrian princes, and of many of the German states.

There are also professors of homeopathy in the University of Prague, of Zurich, of Gallicia, of Christiania, of Munich, of Belgium, of Vienna, Genoa, Naples,

Padoue, Rouen, Boulogne, Valenza, Montpellier, Strasburg, Trieste, Madrid, Coïmbra, Edinburgh, St. Andrew's, and of many medical schools.

There are physicians practising homeopathy in one or more hospitals in the cities of Vienna, Berlin, St. Petersburg, Moscow, Genoa, Valencia, Naples, Rouen, Paris, Marseilles, Madrid, Lisbon, Plainpalais, and many other places; and among the people of every state or country in Europe homeopathy stands higher to-day than at any other time of its history. And the physicians to the families and institutions above mentioned are mostly converts from old school doctrines, embracing men of the very highest order of intellect and acquirements.

Lastly. "Not many years can pass away before the same curiosity excited by one of Perkins's tractors will be awakened at the sight of one of the 'infinitesimal globules.'" "If it should claim a longer existence, it can only be by falling into the hands of the sordid wretches who wring their bread from the cold grasp of disease and death, in the hovels of ignorant poverty." O my!

Twenty-seven years ago pure globules, prepared for medication, were imported by the pound; now they are made in this country, and sold by the hundred, if not by the ton. And is it from sordid wretches, of ignorant poverty, such as passed before the seer's vision, that the forty homeopathic physicians are getting their living in Boston? So far from it is the fact, that it is believed that nearly one half of the wealth is in the hands of homeopathists, and, if we except physicians, more than half of the literary and professional talent. And more than twenty-five years after this lugubrious prophecy, some of us heard this same seer publicly charging the Governor of our Commonwealth with being guilty of placing his valuable life in the hands of homeopathy.

Hahnemann's Ghost.

Thus ends the story of the first valiant attack, in which homeopathy is not only ignominiously killed, but shockingly dismembered. But Banquo's ghost never was half so troublesome to poor Macbeth as has since been the ghost of Hahnemann to our Professor. It not only *gets into his chair* at public dinners, but into his *medical chair*, and at his "Breakfast Table;" —wherever he is, up comes this phantom to plague him, till we can say, as the Salem Register said of the phantom of old John Brown and the Editor of the Boston Courier, We are afraid that poor old Hahnemann, "who is dead and gone, will yet be the death of him."

A New Crusade.

Thus, in 1841, was inaugurated the crusade against homeopathy in New England; and you have had specimens of the "calm investigations" (!) before which it was to succumb in a single hour. But homeopathy "wouldn't stay killed." And many a time, in the twenty-seven years that have since transpired, our modern Macbeth has probably said, in sadness, —

> "The times have been,
> That when the brains were out the man would die,
> And there an end; but now they rise again,
> With twenty mortal murders on their crowns,
> *And push us from our stools:* This is more strange
> Than such a murder is."

Wherever he is, this phantom is at his elbow to torment him. If he sits as "Autocrat of the Breakfast Table," the goblin of Hahnemann and homeopathy are there; and as boys whistle in going by a graveyard, to show they are not afraid, so, to show how little is feared from them, some joke is every day cracked at their expense. And then at medical lectures, — although the subjects are anatomy and physiology — subjects, it might be supposed, not particularly connected with homeopathy, — still, for more than twenty years, poor Hahnemann must always be dragged from his grave to help illustrate them. Lately, however, it is said, he is suffered to rest, as it is not found to be profitable to put the students to thinking about homeopathy. They are sure to come out homeopathists, and in this way the ranks of homeopathic physicians have been mostly supplied.

It would be amusing to give a "history of the crusades" against homeopathy for the last twenty years; but, to do the subject justice, it would require the pen of a Cervantes. Having failed to exterminate it by "a single hour of calm investigation," (!) and having forgotten his promise to "treat it, not by ridicule, but by argument," and for twenty years having applied that means of trying to stop its career, with manifest effect on his students quite different from his expectation, and having succeeded no better with the device of refusing to meet in consultation with old students, calling them quacks, &c., our Harvard Professor found it necessary to call in help to get up a new crusade on a new plan.

We have already referred to the plan of extermination, by refusing to consult with us; but, that failing, we have been not a little amused at another device still more ridiculous. This plan was first made public in 1859, when, after a year of preparation, the Berkshire Professor brought out his big gun.*

After acknowledging the impotence of other persecutions, he says, "I would expel them as quacks." (The cream of this joke consists in the fact that very few of us attend their meetings or take an interest in their proceedings. They can expel us from the privilege of paying three dollars a year for a dinner which we never eat, that is all.) But what is a quack? An ignorant pretender? That won't do, for most of them graduated at our colleges, and none of them pretend to knowledge which they are not willing to communicate to the whole world. Well, a definition must be had that will hit them. "The essence of quackery is, ignoring the wisdom and guidance of the past, and assuming and advertising to be possessed of a skill beyond our con-

* Address by Dr. Timothy Child, of Pittsfield, May 20, 1859.

temporaries." But can't the Doctor see who stands in the range of this shot?

Our Professor so far "ignores the wisdom and guidance of the past," as to propose to throw into the sea almost the entire Materia Medica, which has been accumulating for over two thousand years. And he assumes and advertises a skill in the cure of typhoid fever, that not one of his contemporaries ever dreamed of. And Louis — a name which the Doctor says he can't mention but with profound respect — is also a consummate quack, for he ignores all wisdom, past and present, and sets up a system of his own; and Hunter, Harvey, Newton, Galileo, and old Hippocrates himself, are all quacks, and, according to this definition, *worse* quacks than Hahnemann or any of his disciples.

"His gun, well aimed at duck or plover,
Bears wide and knocks its owner over."

After the address, the Society met and passed a vote of thanks to Dr. Timothy Child, "for his able, interesting, and instructive address;" but not a word is said about carrying out his suggestions. They voted, however, to appoint Dr. Oliver W. Holmes as orator for the next year, thus bringing out their most experienced engineer, to bring to bear his biggest ordnance, and sweep us off forever. And this is the origin of the famous address entitled "Currents and Counter Currents in Medical Science." And when the year came round, didn't we laugh, when instead of an "infernal machine," to scatter us to the four winds, all we got was a few squibs, and *they* mostly aimed at the Professor's own little "pedicular" effigy, while a big bombshell was thrown into his own camp, to blow them all sky high!

Rational Medicine was of course incensed at being thus shown up, and at the meeting of the Massachusetts Medical Society, held as usual on the day of the annual address, for the purpose of voting to print it, an exciting discussion occurred as to the expediency of publishing sentiments so adapted to undermine the confidence of the public in their mode of practice; but its publication was finally determined on, upon the ground that suppressing the truth was more dangerous than the truth itself.

The last act in this interesting drama, to which I shall refer, relates to

The City Hospital in Boston.

In 1864 a Hospital was opened for the benefit of that class of people who, when well, are able to provide for themselves, but when sick, are destitute, and dependent on others. It is supported by taxation, and, of course, all holders of property share alike in its burdens. Before it was opened, a petition was presented to the trustees, signed by eight hundred of our most influential tax-payers, embracing senators, members of congress, judges, lawyers, clergymen, editors, capitalists, and all other classes of our most intelligent and influential citizens, in the following words: —

"The undersigned, citizens of Boston, respectfully represent, that while a large part of our intelligent inhabitants believe that the homeopathic method of curing diseases is the safest, quickest, and most reliable, and therefore employ no other in their families, there is not in Boston a place where the stranger and the homeless can enjoy its advantages. We therefore request that a part of the City Hospital may be devoted to the practice of homeopathy, under regulations which shall secure the same privileges as other patients enjoy."

Of these petitioners, the large majority were gentlemen known to be believers of homeopathy, and to practise it exclusively in their families; but to test public sentiment, an application for signatures was made to two hundred in one ward, and one hundred in another, of the principal citizens, by individuals ignorant of their opinions on the subject; and of these three hundred voters, only six refused to sign, and they only on the ground of personal relations to old school doctors.

And instead of eight hundred signatures, there might have been obtained those of all the respectable citizens in Boston, except the old school doctors and a few of their personal friends — all seeing and acknowledging the justice of the request.

With this petition was presented a memorial, showing by statistics, facts, and arguments, the claims of homeopathy to the confidence of the community. It was kindly received by the trustees, and its claims fully discussed; and, not one of them being controverted, and all the principal newspapers, as well as every influential citizen, acknowledging their justice, they gave us assurance, as far as individual opinion could go, that our request would be granted.

But when appointments of physicians came to be made, it was found that the old school physicians had clubbed together to keep out homeopathists, and had resolved that they would accept of no appointment if any homeopathists should be appointed, even though they might be graduates with them, at their own medical school; thus driving the trustees to the alternative of excluding homeopathists, or giving up the establishment to them exclusively. And the result is, that homeopathists, who pay nearly if not quite half the expenses, are expelled from the hospital, or, what is worse, if they go there, are obliged to take crude drugs which they heartily abhor; and whether they take them or not, are obliged to pay thousands of dollars every year for drugs, spirits, beers, and hospital stores, ninety per cent. of which they religiously believe are worse than useless.

When the medical spirit that thus sacrifices the interests of our best citizens to the hatred of fellow-graduates of the same school, for no other reason than that, following the dictates of reason and conscience, they have adopted a system of cure vastly superior to their own, shall be looked upon by the medical light of the twentieth century, as we now look back on the religious bigotry that whipped Quakers and banished Baptists by the religious light of the nineteenth, this item of history may be interesting.

I therefore make a record of the ingenious way by which, without controverting a statement, or answering an argument of the petitioners, through their Doctor on the Board they contrive to take possession of the hospital, and exclude other doctors who were educated with them. And, that I may not misrepresent them, I give the report of the Doctor on the subject verbatim.

"The undersigned, to whom was referred the subject of the introduction of Homeopathic Medical Practice into the City Hospital, have examined with care the various documents submitted to them. These documents consist of —

"1. A petition signed by eight hundred citizens of Boston, accompanied by a Memorial, containing arguments and statistics, by Albert J. Bellows, M. D.

"2. A letter from the same gentleman, dated January 12, 1864.

"3. A communication from the Boston Academy of Homeopathic Medicine, dated May 27, 1863.

"4. A letter signed by seven physicians of the Homeopathic Medical Dispensary.

"5. A communication from J. T. Talbot, M. D., dated June 1, 1863.

"In document No. 1 the petitioners ask that 'a part of the City Hospital may be devoted to the practice of homeopathy, under regulations which shall secure the same privileges as other patients enjoy.'

"In No. 2 the same request is made, and the writer

asks that he may be appointed Medical Director and Attending Physician to that department, 'according to the nomination of the Boston Academy, composed of about forty physicians, all of whom are regularly educated, and most of them graduates of allopathic colleges.'

"Document No. 3 contains the proceedings of a meeting of the Boston Academy of Homeopathic Medicine, at which the following conclusions were unanimously decided upon, namely:—

"'In order to give homeopathic science a just trial, it would be necessary to place the department under the medical direction of some member of our branch of the profession, who has the confidence of his fellows as being capable of doing justice to such a responsible station; and that, independently of all other medical influence, he should have charge of the preparation of medicines, the charge of the nurses, and of everything else pertaining to the treatment of patients in his department; and that, in order to accomplish this successfully, he must reside in the hospital.

"'They also recommend the appointment of a Board of Visiting Physicians, including, at least, one competent and experienced surgeon, who have confidence in the medical director and each other.' A committee of three was appointed to nominate such a board to be recommended to the Hospital. It was also voted unanimously 'that we recommend the appointment of Albert J. Bellows, M. D., as Medical Director and Attending Physician of the Homeopathic Department of the Free City Hospital, under such arrangements as shall be satisfactory to him, and shall secure to such patients as shall prefer our method of treatment the benefit of humane and careful attendance, and the scientific administration of curative agents.'

"Paper No. 4 is signed by seven gentlemen, physicians of the Homeopathic Medical Dispensary, and dwells upon the benefits derived by certain classes by the establishment of a City Hospital, and requests that the classes alluded to may be allowed the privilege of placing themselves therein under homeopathic treatment.

"No. 5 is a communication from a medical practitioner upon the feasibility of introducing the system of homeopathic treatment into the new City Hospital. It quotes instances, from personal observation during the years 1853-1854, where the two systems of treatment had been successfully introduced under the same management, or into the same building. Such instances were witnessed by the writer at Bremen, at Linz, at Vienna, and at the Hospitals of Saint Marguerite and Beaujou in Paris.

"The Board of Trustees have, during the past year, granted hearings to parties representing different opinions in regard to the subject contained in the documents above referred to, and are therefore equally well informed with the Committee as to the various arguments in the case.

"Your Committee do not feel that you have intrusted them with the duty of deciding upon the merits of the two modes of medical treatment which it is proposed to introduce into the hospital; nor would they feel competent to such a task, had the duty been assigned them. They have endeavored, in their inquiries, to confine themselves to the simple, practical question, whether the admission to the Hospital of two opposing modes of treatment, and two classes of practitioners, would conduce to the prosperity of the institution or the welfare of its inmates. On the score of humanity, it would seem most desirable that each beneficiary of this noble charity should be followed to its wards, and receive the care of the physicians of his choice, whether he were a believer in the homeopathic, the hydropathic, the botanic, or the spiritual system of medical treatment. Each has its numerous advocates and practitioners; and if one be admitted without reference to any standard, could the others be consistently excluded?

"We do not doubt the intelligence of the class of patients for whose benefit the Hospital has been established. They are not to be the paupers of the city, but persons who can, in health, support themselves by their own industry. How many of them when taken sick would, if left to themselves, think of the method of treatment to which they would be subjected? We think there would be very few. They would submit themselves, with readiness, to the kind attentions and skill of those who command the confidence of a vast majority in the community, and who worthily represent the medical profession, in all its progress and advancement, as it has existed for many centuries.

"It can readily be seen what effect would be produced upon the management and discipline of the institution, should there be an indiscriminate admission of practitioners who would owe no responsibility to the trustees, and who could not be subjected to their control. If an exception should now be made in favor of the petitioners, we cannot see, with the present disposition of the buildings, how such an arrangement would be carried out.

"So far as we can learn, the instances quoted of similar arrangements in Europe would not afford encouragement for the experiment here. The hospital at Vienna, we are informed by a gentleman who visited that city within a few months, is a small establishment, entirely distinct, and in a remote part of the city. Government in Austria assumes the control of almost every institution, and it is, therefore, under the same management as the Grand Hospital, containing two thousand six hundred beds, in another part of the city. It is patronized principally by a few wealthy persons in the community.

"The hospital at Linz is also a distinctly homeopathic institution. The hospital at Bremen, at least that part devoted to the homeopathic treatment, has been discontinued. Of the Saint Marguerite, at Paris, we have no definite information. Our informant visited the Beaujou very recently, but neither saw nor heard anything of the arrangement which existed in 1854. Whether this be so or not, the fact mentioned in document No. 5, above quoted, of the remonstrance to the director-general by other physicians, on account of the innovations, proves that the plan did not tend to harmony in management.

"Your petitioners affirm, in document No. 3, 'that, in order to give homeopathic science a just trial, a medical director should have exclusive control of the ward assigned to them, and should reside in the Hospital.' It can easily be seen what would be the result of such a plan, when we remember that, by Section 4 of the City Ordinance, creating the Hospital, it is provided that the superintendent 'shall have, under the trustees, the control of *all* departments of the Hospital; of all subordinate officers, attendants, domestics; of the patients; and the charge of the grounds, buildings, and appurtenances.'

"With the present limited number of buildings at our disposal, and the divisions made necessary for the accommodation of male and female medical and surgical patients, your Committee can see no way by which the wishes of the very respectable body of petitioners can be complied with; and they have, furthermore, sufficient faith in their intelligence to believe that, when all the facts stated are reviewed, they will see the impracticability of the plan which they have proposed. For the still more potent reason that such a scheme would be fatal to the harmony necessary to the full success and usefulness of the new Hospital, they recommend that no departure be made from the rules which prevail on this subject in other kindred institutions.

(Signed) WM. R. LAWRENCE, SUMNER CROSBY, } *Committee.*

"BOSTON, Jan. 23, 1864."

The Report, it will be seen, is mostly occupied with a communication from the Boston Academy of Homeopathic Medicine, dated May 27, 1863, suggesting the necessity of having a resident homeopathic physician, &c.

These suggestions were made under the impression, received from the Chairman of the Board, that a resident old school physician would be appointed. And I only consented to think of accepting their nomination, and go into the Hospital, if elected, upon condition that it should prove to be the only way in which to accomplish an object worthy of such a sacrifice.

But when the application was made, knowing the plan of having a resident physician had been abandoned, and expecting the subject would be committed to one desirous of trying to make it practicable to grant our petition, — that being the opinion of a majority of the members, — I simply suggested that the request of the Academy should be so modified as to make it practicable under existing circumstances. The subject was, however, called up by, and of course committed to a physician, who, very naturally, favored the wishes of his old school brethren; and, ignoring my suggestion for modification, he devoted most of his Report to the proof that the suggestions of the Academy were inconsistent with the arrangements of the Hospital, and impracticable, and therefore he could "see no way by which the wishes of the very respectable body of petitioners can be complied with."

The Report proves, I acknowledge, conclusively, that

it was inconsistent to grant the petitioners what they did *not desire* to have, and that question was settled. And I asked the Board to consider whether it proved it to be inconsistent, or impracticable, to grant us what we *did want*, under the arrangements then made. What we really did desire, was simply this: that the superintendent be authorized to furnish accommodations, at his own discretion, for such patients as preferred homeopathic treatment, and that, under their rules and ordinances, and subject to all of them, they should appoint such medical attendance for them as was necessary to give them appropriate homeopathic treatment; but that they should appoint no one who could not come in under the same standard as that under which their other appointments were made.

The very statement of this question knocked out the principal pillars on which the conclusion rested, that our petition should not be granted. The argument, as seen by the Doctor's report, is thus stated: "The homeopathic, the hydropathic, the botanic, and the spiritual systems of medical treatment, each has its numerous advocates and practitioners, and if one be admitted, without reference to any standard, could the others be consistently excluded?" But we claimed to come in under their own standard. What was the standard by which they appointed the Board of Physicians already chosen? Had they all a diploma from some accredited medical college? So had we, and mostly from the very same. If that was not the standard, it would not be easy to name one that could admit all the physicians already chosen and exclude us. Did we differ from them in mode of practice? So did they differ from one another. Let us illustrate: —

Three patients are sick alike. One wants a doctor who will do something, and they have for him the heroic practitioner, who would bleed him, and blister him, and torment him generally, to his full satisfaction. The second preferred to dispense with such luxuries, and they had for him the expectant practitioner, who would carefully see to his nursing and diet, and the air he breathes, &c., but would give him no medicine. The third would like a treatment exactly like the second, but would like, in addition, some homeopathic globules, and asked for a doctor who graduated with the other two, and agreed with both in regard to general management, diet, &c., and differed from the second only in what relates to the homeopathic globules.

They appoint the two first-mentioned practitioners, but when the third is nominated, "a horrid spectre rises to their sight, close by their side, and plain and palpable," threatening to slip in; and lest it might succeed, they shut the door on goblin and doctor together.

But was it fair or just to shut out, among the quacks, that doctor who had not the slightest affinity for them, while those were admitted whose therapeutics are, by their own admission, very nearly allied to theirs?

I will quote the opinions on this subject of some of the most learned men in the world. Professor Broussais, who is styled the illustrious Professor of Val de Grace, says, "I agree that medicine has rendered to suffering man the service of offering him consolations, by ever fostering chimerical hopes; but such service is far from placing it on a level with other natural sciences. It rather seems to class it with astrology, superstition, and all kinds of quackery." Professor Magendie, whose writings are in the libraries of all respectable physicians, says, "It is especially where medicine is most active that mortality is greatest." And the learned Professor of Harvard Medical College, whose advice was had on the question of admitting homeopathy, says, "The truth is, that medicine, professedly founded on observation, is as sensitive to outside influences, political, religious, philosophical, and imaginary, as is the barometer to atmospheric density."

The most celebrated physicians and professors in the hospitals in Paris — Valleix, Fodera, Bichat, Rostan, Louis, Chomel, Bouchardat, and Calvi — have all expressed similar sentiments respecting the absolute worthlessness of the allopathic systems of *materia medica*. While on the other hand, men equally learned agree that the system of homeopathic therapeutics is founded on an immutable law of Nature.

Marchal de Calvi, the learned professor already mentioned, says, "There is nothing satisfactory in teaching *materia medica* according to the approved system." "All we know of any value about it, we owe to the works of homeopathists." "In the works of physicians of the lawful school, from Hippocrates downward to our times, we find absolutely nothing."

Professor Gourboyer says, "All researches of scholars

confirm on every point the therapeutical truths taught by Hahnemann." "The more I study the works of different schools, the more I am astonished at the conclusions in favor of homeopathy." "I challenge all honest and intelligent physicians, who will faithfully examine all systems and works of *materia medica*, to arrive at a different conclusion." Scores of other men, equally learned, will give similar testimony, corroborating these statements; and yet the Report persists in consigning us to the company of quacks outside their institution, while those thus proved to be more allied to them are admitted, and our patients are expected to submit to their treatment without a question. In what respect do we not "represent the medical profession in all its progress and advancement as it has existed for many centuries," according to their own standard?

But the most potent reason for rejecting our petition is, that "it would be fatal to the harmony necessary to the full success and usefulness of the new Hospital." And how was this terrible evil to be produced by the introduction of homeopathy? Two classes of regular physicians were already appointed, as we have seen, so that it would follow that while one patient was bled, and blistered, and took blue pill, another, with the same disease, might be permitted to die a natural death, or get well with good nursing, without medicine.

Now the innovation we proposed to make, was to add to the treatment of the expectant patient perhaps the millionth of a grain of aconite every hour or two, or something else equally formidable; and this was the enemy that would be fatal to the harmony of the Institution. The contest then was between the old school doctors and the infinitesimal globule which they so affected to despise.

The next reason for rejecting our petition was, that so far as the committee could see, "the instances quoted of similar arrangements in Europe would not afford encouragement for the experiment here."

When that sentence was written, there was in the hands of the committee our Memorial, and two pamphlets corroborating it, referring to more than a score of hospitals in which homeopathy had been successfully and harmoniously tried in connection with old school practice, or under the same control.

In this Memorial it was also asserted and proved that old school practitioners and homeopathists differ only in the administration of medicine, and in that even differ less from some of them than they differ from each other, and that, therefore, nothing would prevent harmony but the opposition of these physicians; and this had always proved to be the truth.

We also stated, and proved by statistics, that homeopathy saves fifty per cent. more of life than the other school; that it saves more than one quarter of the time, and therefore of the expenses, of the patients; that it saves the terrible sufferings from lancets, blisters, caustics, and poisonous drugs, and the diseases entailed by them; and these facts and statements, and many more, had been presented to the Professor of Harvard Medical

School, who for twenty-seven years had made homeopathy his specialty, with the request that, after carefully considering them, he would go before the trustees and point out their errors and defects, if such could be found.

For a fortnight the learned Professor did give special attention to the subject, as his students testify, as also to the fact that in his researches for the cause and cure of homeopathy, and the reason for failure in his former attempts to rid medical science of this its direst pest, he had discovered that all this time he had mistaken its entomological character, classing it with humbugs, when in fact it belonged to a very different class of vermin.

The important discovery was not divulged to his class till the very day on which he was to administer his exterminating *enema*, and then in these words: "These pestilent homeopathists give me immense trouble." "They are the Ascarides in the rectum of medical science." "And I have an appointment to meet the Trustees of the new Hospital, and help expel them."

He did meet with them, and passed three or four hours; and his attention was frequently called to the statements and statistics of the Memorial; but he neither corrected nor disputed a single one of them. Now, if there had been misstatements, or errors of statistics, it is certain that he would have made an *enema* of them like a "clyster of fish-hooks," if I may be allowed to carry out the classical and poetical figure of this celebrated author and poet. Think you that, with such means of exterminating us, he would have spent three precious hours in descanting on such subjects as the appropriate homeopathic remedies for sneezing and hiccough, or portraying the evils that would come from tying cats' tails together, and throwing them over a clothes-line?

All the statements in the Memorial, then, were true; and yet, ignoring all this proof to the contrary, the Doctor takes a single statement from another document, that at one time certain physicians petitioned the governor-general of the hospitals in Paris to have the homeopathic doctor removed; and makes that prove that "such arrangements do not tend to harmony," and there "is no encouragement for the experiment here."

As this is all the proof he offers, let us examine the case, and see how much it proves. The facts are these: —

In 1849, M. Tessier, by virtue of his superior abilities and acquirements, and not as a homeopathist, was assigned a ward in Saint Marguerite Hospital, in Paris. He believed in homeopathy, and therefore practised it. In 1851 it came to be known that the mortality, length of disease, and expense in his ward were much less than in the other wards. This fact excited among the doctors of the baser sort a spirit of jealousy, and they circulated slanders against him, and grossly misrepresented the results of his practice, and even tried to counteract the effects of his medicine by fumigation, &c., and finally raised a committee to report to the governor-general that homeopathy did not tend to harmony — was a total failure, &c., and that Dr. Tessier ought to be removed. The governor-general, seeing through the plot, sent the slanderers to their own place in the dark; and Tessier remained there, and in the Beaujou, under the same control, for thirteen years, till 1862, when he died, having established the claims of homeopathy in the minds of the most intelligent people of Paris beyond a doubt. And, though he suffered much from the slanders of the lowest order of physicians, up to the day of his death he had the confidence and friendship of the most learned of his profession, and for the last year of his life was physician to the Empress Eugenie. And this is the case about which, after diligent search, nothing could be found, but which proves to the mind of the Committee that, at any rate, "the plan did not tend to harmony."

They did find, however, two small hospitals in Austria, and also learned that the one at Bremen had been given up, leaving on your minds, whether intentional or not, the impression that homeopathy in Europe is confined to two or three small establishments, and that even in them it is dying out.

That this impression was wrong, we have seen by statistics already given; and as for the harmony, it was true that up to 1853 or 1854, in one sense, the introduction of homeopathy into a hospital or college did not tend to harmony — that is, allopathic physicians made such a fuss as to cause great disturbance, and, in some instances, to succeed in driving off the non-combative homeopathist; but in no other way has harmony ever been disturbed; and since then there has really been comparatively little disturbance, especially among the better classes of physicians, who almost universally recognize the claims of homeopathy as an exact science.

The Doctor thought that of the intelligent patients, for whose benefit the hospital was established, very few, when taken sick, would think of the treatment to which they would be subjected. If this had proved to be true, the beds would have been spared for other patients, as he desired, and the community would have been satisfied, as a choice of treatment would have been offered them.

But what do facts indicate in the case? I knew, and probably every other homeopathic physician knew, of cases of boarders, or seamstresses, or servants, who were being cared for under great disadvantages, and who would have been very glad of beds in the hospital, but who would have died in an attic alone rather than go there to take crude medicines. And we know of ladies now who take care of their servants, and do their work for them, rather than have them exposed to such treatment. The Doctor had no conception of the horror a genuine homeopathist has of crude drugs.

Another serious difficulty was expressed as follows: "With the present limited number of buildings at our disposal, and the divisions made necessary for the accommodation of male and female medical and surgical patients, your Committee can see no way by which the wishes of the very respectable body of petitioners can be complied with." There were, besides the six large wards that have room for twenty-eight beds in each, many others of all sizes, from a single bed to seven beds. And we offered to show to any committee, that all we asked could be given us without the slightest inconvenience to any arrangements. But suppose it had been inconvenient to grant the request of the petitioners, should they, for that reason, have ignored the claims of citizens who pay one third of the expenses? It certainly was inconvenient for them to be shut out.

Let us look at the ethics of this question through a simple illustration. Three brothers build a house to live in, *à la* Hotel Pelham, each paying equal shares. When it is done, it is found that the families of A and B are so prejudiced against the family of C that they study how not to let him in. A says to B, Our families are large, and we can find use for all the rooms ourselves. We are conservative, and want to continue the good old customs taught by our fathers for centuries, and handed down to us. We used to take brimstone every other day, and have the colic as often, and when we got over it always felt better; and, being alive yet, we cherish the old system, and wish to transmit it to our children. But C has a crotchet in his head that colic is unwholesome, and he uses brimstone only in homeopathic doses.

Now, it will readily be seen that, if his children get along without brimstone and the colic, our children will want to dispense with them also, and that would be fatal to harmony. The thing was tried in France once, and that was the result. Besides, if our brother comes in, some loafer will want to come in with him. Now let us tell C: he is a very respectable young man, and intelligent withal, and will see at once the force of our argument, especially as two is a large majority against one, and majorities are expected to control personal rights. His family is small, and needs but little room, and is, therefore, indifferent about *any;* and, under these circumstances, we propose to take all the rooms ourselves, and, after we are fairly settled, perhaps we may find a room sufficiently isolated to be safe, or, what would be better, perhaps, build him a cottage by himself. But C answers, We can't see the point. Small as we are, we feel the cold outside, and know our rights within. Still, being small and good-natured, we only ask for a little room till we grow to need more. Is this unreasonable?

Having followed the Doctor's suggestions, and reviewed all the facts presented, we came to conclusions differing widely from those of the Report. Nor could we agree with it, that it was best to start the concern before this question was settled. We thought the best time to get into the cars was before they had started; and, therefore, asked the Board to take up the petition again, and give it to a committee, with instructions to report whether homeopathy might not be introduced, in accordance with the wishes of the petitioners, and the wishes of the community, as expressed in all the public journals, and yet in accordance with all the rules and ordinances of the institution. Of course it did not comport with the wishes of the doctors who controlled the matter to have it reconsidered; and, notwithstanding the wishes of the community, and the positive proof that homeopathy not only cuts short diseases, but increases the chances of life, — facts so fully understood that some of the best insurance companies will insure the lives of those who allow no other practice for fifteen per cent. less than others, — yet, for four years, the Hospital has been carried on under the exclusive direction of old school physicians, the good-natured homeopathists paying half of the enormous expenses.

But if they *enjoy* the monopoly, certainly homeopathic physicians have no reason to complain, for the facts to which I have referred having been brought out by the discussion, and the community seeing, as they never saw before, the real merits of the new system, are rapidly embracing it; and the number of homeopathic physicians in Boston, in the mean time, has increased more than one third, being now over fifty, while in 1864 it was less than thirty.

And if we are the ignorant quacks we are charged with being, we are ignorant in spite of all the knowledge we could get from Harvard Medical College, being mostly graduates from that institution; and although it requires three times as many families to support us as it does to support our allopathic brethren, our patients being sick but half as long, and less than half as often as theirs, we are all getting a good living. So that, for the next Act in this interesting Drama we can afford to wait, and, attending to our own business, imitate the example of the good-natured husband, who cheerfully submitted to the tirade of his little wife, because it did him no harm, and seemed to do her so much good.

MEDICINES A GIFT FROM GOD.

Nothing in Nature exhibits to my mind more clearly the benevolence of God, than his provision for relieving sufferings by medicine. If these sufferings were inevitable, even human benevolence might, if possible, provide a remedy; but being the result — as every one of them is — of some breach of some clearly-revealed law, it seems nothing short of a miracle of mercy that in the noisome weed at our door, in the fang of the serpent, in the sting of the bee, in the mineral poisons, as well as in the beautiful plants and flowers of the field, there should be provided, beforehand, "a balm for every wound," — a relief for every pain.

But nothing can be more clearly proved than that such a provision is made, even for sufferings which we can trace directly to imprudences and sins. A man imprudently exposes himself to wet and cold, and, in consequence, his tonsils swell, fever comes on, and he is prostrated with sickness. He takes of deadly nightshade and wasp-bane, — two of our most poisonous weeds, — in divided doses too small to do the slightest harm, and is cured perhaps in a single night.

Or he eats imprudently, and colic is induced, and he takes perhaps the hundredth part of a drop of the tincture of nux vomica, and is relieved, it may be, in ten minutes.

Or he takes improper food and drinks, and his blood becomes low, and dropsical deposits are gathered, to the amount, it may be, of gallons, and a medicine prepared from the sting of a single bee may remove it in three weeks, although it might have been months in accumulating.

Or he wickedly contracts some disease, which is cured perfectly by inoffensive doses of mineral medicine.

Or he has an old sore, that has lasted for years, and has resisted corrosive, caustic, and all sorts of harsh medicines; but the application of tea, made from a common plant, may heal it perfectly.

These are but the recitation of influences that come daily under the observation of all homeopathic physicians, and prove to my mind conclusively that this is Nature's plan for curing diseases.

Crude Drugs Dangerous.

If it be true that such simple means are all that are required to remove the gravest diseases, — and nothing can be more clearly proved, — surely it is important that the fact should be known, especially to mothers; for however otherwise doctors may differ, they all agree in this: that castor oil, rhubarb, Ayer's pills, and all kinds of cathartics, and other active medicines, do immense injury to the constitution, causing, as they do, much of the temporary suffering from constipation, hemorrhoids, colics, liver complaints, dyspepsia, &c., from which, in the way in which most mothers manage their children, very few are exempt, and perpetuating these sufferings during all their lives.

And in view of these opinions, corroborated as they are by the facts presented in the chapter on the Uses and Abuses of Medicines, every intelligent doctor, not only, but, on reflection, every intelligent man and woman, would join me in advice to every family in the country and the world, as the first step towards securing their families from attacks of sickness and pain, and towards giving their children a chance to live and enjoy health, to banish from the house, and never again allow to enter it, every bottle and package of castor oil, rhubarb, pills, soothing syrup, paregoric, patent medicine, and every other crude article of medicine.

It is a matter of common observation, that those families who resort, at every attack of colic, or pain from indigestion, or any other derangement of the digestive organs, to rhubarb, or elixir pro, or pain-killer, or any other drug which affords relief, have a constant use for them, and, if the dose taken is large, the more sure the relief the more certain the recurrence of disease. Now this fact is not only in accordance with experience and observation, but it is in accordance with the law of Nature, which I have elsewhere explained, given on purpose to show us what a medicine will do, and thus show us what symptoms it will relieve.

Take for example, Brandreth's pills, which for the last fifty years have been perhaps the sovereign remedy in more families in this country than any other compound. Their principal ingredients are aloes and colocynth — medicines which form the basis of almost all the drastic pills which have been used for the last fifty years, as pill cochiac, pill rufi, Ayer's pills, &c., which almost always produce colics and pains, and which have probably been the cause of more piles, dysenteries, and liver complaints, a thousand times over, than they ever cured.

These medicines do undoubtedly relieve pain for the time, as, when a boy, I had occasion to know by experience; but, as I also fully remember, those pains would soon return: and thus for weeks together no day would pass without a resort to this, or some other abominable drug. The first attack was probably caused by some indigestible food; all the others by the pills which were taken to cure it.

That both aloes and colocynth will cause indigestion, colics, piles, and other troubles, has been proved a hundred times over — not only by observing the effects of pills, so universally used, but by careful proving of them by persons in health. And there is not a doubt in the minds of those who have investigated the subject, that ninety-nine hundredths of all the sickness and suffering of those who habitually resort to active crude drugs for relief of pain, are caused and perpetuated by the very drugs to which they resort.

If that be true, ninety-nine hundredths of all their sufferings would be saved by banishing, and placing beyond their reach, all such drugs and medicines.

Without such precaution, it would be in vain to resolve not to use these deleterious articles, for, when a child is sick, the mother will instinctively do something for its relief; and, in a sudden and violent attack of pain, I have known mothers kill their children outright with opium, or antimony, or even arsenic, in their thoughtless desperation. How vastly important, then, that mothers should study to know what to do in case of sickness, and be prepared to do it, otherwise, though she may not be in great danger of killing her children outright, there is certainly a probability, in the present state of ignorance in the community on that subject, of doing harm rather than good, even if she have no deleterious drugs in her own house.

In this case the child will take, of course, what the nearest neighbor happens to have.

If pain-killer, or composition, or any other of those violent stimulants recommended by that class of practitioners who, though they have a horror of mineral medicines, give vegetable poisons much more virulent, down will go into the delicate stomach enough to draw a blister, or inflame a surface of the skin, if applied outside, of many inches in extent.

If paregoric, soothing syrup, or laudanum, down will go enough of that to make it stupid for twenty-four hours.

If Ayer's Pills, or Mandrake Pills, or any other of the popular cathartic medicines, down will go enough of aloes, colocynth, or podophylon, to lay the foundation of piles, colics, dyspepsias, and liver complaints,

— if followed up after the usual fashion, — that will last the lifetime.

And thus are laid the foundations of much of the suffering in community; and so persistent are ignorant and reckless neighbors in the idea that whatever they have used, especially if their mother used it before them, — even if half their children had died under its use, — is the best and only thing to be used in any sickness, that in some neighborhoods, while a doctor, whose business it is to give what is best and avoid everything else, is paid for regular attendance, a child cannot be sick a week till some neighbor shall insist on smuggling into it, without the doctor's knowledge, their own sovereign remedy.

I once had a family of four children sick at once with scarlet fever. They were all very sick; but, under proper treatment, I expected they would all recover — as they did. When they were sickest, a woman came some miles from the country, not knowing the afflicted mother, but hearing of the sickness of her children. She said she felt great sympathy for her, for she had experienced the same trial, having had four children sick at once with the same disease; and having heard of her afflictions she had come down to do what she could for her.

She had, she said, an excellent medicine, which she always used in case of sickness, and her mother used it before her, and it always did good, and was perfectly harmless. (This last merit, by the way, pertains to all domestic and quack medicines, however virulent: in the opinion of their advocate, they are always harmless.) She said she gave it to her children between the doctor's doses, and it did them a great deal of good.

She was asked how long her children were sick. "O, not very long. They got along nicely for about a week, and then they suddenly got worse, — she never could tell why, — and three of them died; but the other got well, and is now the smartest boy in the neighborhood." The afflicted mother concluded not to try the medicine, and after the children were better, she told me the story as I have recorded it.

If a young mother has no fixed opinions respecting the uses and abuses of medicines, the prospect of raising her child, and securing for it any degree of comfort and health, depends very much on her neighbors; and she may bless God for the providence that shall place her in a homeopathic neighborhood. And this brings me to the consideration of

The Importance of Fixed Principles in Medicine.

The medical world may be divided, so far as relates to the use of medicine, into three classes: 1. *Heroic Practitioners* — Those who use crude and poisonous medicines. 2. *Expectant Practitioners* — Those who trust to Nature, and use no medicine. 3. *Homeopathists* — Those who use homeopathic medicine.

Heroic Treatment of Disease.

Those who believe in and depend on crude, active, poisonous medicines for the cure of disease, are styled *heroic* practitioners. Of this class the celebrated Dr. Benjamin Rush, who commenced his practice in this country one hundred years ago, is a strong representative. So important did he consider medicine in the cure of disease, that he declared it to be his opinion that thousands of patients had been sacrificed by the followers of Hippocrates, "by letting Nature loose upon sick people." This class includes Eclectic practitioners, whose predominant characteristic is that they use no mineral medicines, although they use vegetable medicines equally poisonous, and, some of them, quite as virulent; and it includes also the supporters and consumers of all the quack nostrums with which the world is flooded.

The terrible fault of this class is, they do not understand the medical power of Nature. They do not know that Nature always tries to cure disease, and will generally succeed if not interfered with. But that this is true is abundantly proved, as is also the fact that crude medicines do interfere with Nature's arrangements for cure, and thus cause the death of patients innumerable. For proof of this alarming fact, see quotations already made from the celebrated Professor Magendie, that "it is especially where medicine is most active that mortality is greatest;" see also statistics, recorded page 216, showing that in the best hospitals in Europe a large per cent. of the deaths were sacrifices to crude drugs, and that patients who took no medicine recovered in one third less time than those who took crude medicines. And these were facts established by carefully collected statistics, and they have never, to my knowledge, been controverted or disputed.

Expectant Practitioners.

To this second class belong those who trust mostly to Nature, and are afraid of medicine.

This system of practice was instituted by Hippocrates before the Christian era. He believed that Nature would cure all diseases if not interfered with, and therefore was very careful not to give medicine till the disease was removed; but had a curious idea that Nature needed some help in clearing up the *debris* that remained, and therefore gave medicine when the patient was recovering. But he established a very important fact —

Nature can and does remove very serious diseases without the aid of medicine.

Since the age of Hippocrates, the most common-sense practitioners have been most careful not to interfere with Nature by giving active medicine; still the tendency of the profession has always been to forget the teachings of Hippocrates, and trust to medicine rather than to Nature for cure.

But when, more than fifty years ago, Hahnemann began to teach that doses of medicine exceedingly minute would cure disease, if given according to certain principles which he established, those who remembered the teachings of Hippocrates naturally inferred that the influence that Hahnemann imputed to globules was really the *vis medicatrix naturæ.*

They could not deny the fact that Hahnemann's patients did more of them recover, and that much sooner, than those who were treated heroically. And this inspired more confidence in the medical power of Nature, and they have gradually diminished their medicine, till their practice has come to justify the definition given to the practice by the celebrated French professor, who said, "Medicine is the art of pleasing the patient while Nature cures the disease."

That this *placebo* practice is a vast improvement over that murderous heroic practice still believed in and practised by so many now, even in Boston, — but less here, perhaps, than any other place in the world, — not only in regard to the comfort of the patient, but in the number of recoveries, and length of time required for treatment, is shown by experiments and statistics, from which there can be no appeal.

About forty years ago, Louis, a physician to one of the largest hospitals in Paris, probably instigated by the facts before mentioned relating to the success of Hahnemann, instituted experiments, on a large scale, to test the value of active medicine. He placed side by side, in the same hospital, in separate wards, two hundred patients with the same disease, and, except in regard to medicine, with exactly the same treatment; but to one hundred he gave the usual medicines, and the other hundred he trusted to Nature without medicine.

To the mortification of heroic practitioners, he found that the number of deaths was the largest, and the time of sickness the longest, among those who had the usual treatment of medicine. And this important fact has been established in relation to all classes of diseases by numerous similar experiments, corroborating the statement of Magendie and the statistics already referred to.

These facts are not given to show that the services of rational practitioners are valueless to their patients; for, however difficult it may be to show how a heroic practitioner can give an equivalent for the terrible effects of the crude drugs which he administers, yet the rational practitioner, especially if he is not deluded with the idea that alcohol is nutritious, and that crude, disorganized iron furnishes material for red blood, may and does furnish an equivalent for his fees in the care and general management of the case, and in the confidence inspired by having some one at the helm who is supposed to understand navigating in such storms. Still it is no more clearly proved that rational practice is an improvement on heroic practice than it is proved that homeopathic is an improvement on rational practice.

Homeopathic Treatment of Disease.

The statistics, already referred to, which show that a large per cent. of patients, and much of the time of sickness, are lost by active medicines, compared with those in the same hospitals who have no medicines, show that a larger per cent. of deaths and a larger part of the time of sickness are saved by homeopathic treatment, compared with the expectant or do-nothing treatment. See statistics on page 219. These facts show to unprejudiced minds conclusively, that, besides the exemption from doing harm which homeopathy has in common with expectant treatment, there is an important positive influence of homeopathic medicine in assisting Nature in the removal of disease; and yet expectant practitioners, whose minds are riveted to the idea that "homeopathy is a specious mode of doing nothing," cannot be made to see or acknowledge these undisputed and indisputable facts, and, what is worse, they are a thousand times more bitter against homeopathy and homeopathic physicians, — especially if they graduated, as most of us did, at their colleges, — than are heroic practitioners. And as most people have unbounded confidence in the opinion of their doctor, and as they look to no other source for information respecting this or any other subject pertaining to medicine, they are, of course, kept in ignorance of its real merits.

Of hundreds who have told me what their doctors said of homeopathy, not one of them ever got anything like the truth either in regard to the principles or practice of it; and the ideas thus obtained of it are the most absurd and contradictory.

One tells them it is trusting to Nature, and humbugging the patient with the pretence that sugar globules have some influence in the cure; and to prove that this pretended medicine can do no good, they offer to swallow a whole bottleful. Of the millions of families who have used these globules for years, there is not an intelligent man or woman who does not know that they do have an effect, though they may not understand how it is done. Take, for example, the single article, aconite.

Millions of intelligent people will testify that they have experienced or witnessed, in the case of a burning fever suddenly induced, a sensible influence in cooling it down from globules of aconite, in less than twenty minutes. What folly to attempt to prove to such people, by swallowing a bottleful of globules of aconite, that they have been deceived by their senses and their consciousness!

Besides, the very idea that nothing can do good that cannot do harm, is perfectly heathenish, and contrary to all the laws of Nature, as I have elsewhere shown. There is not, in the whole range of sciences, a single branch established by such an accumulation of facts and experiments as the principles of homeopathy.

That the earth revolves round the sun, and the moon round the earth; that caustic lime and more caustic sulphuric acid will unite to form inert gypsum; that it took ages to construct the earth as we now find it, instead of a single week; and a hundred other similar propositions not more reasonable to the uneducated mind, and not supported by half the facts or arguments as the proposition that any medicinal substance which in large doses will produce certain symptoms will in small doses relieve similar symptoms, are propositions believed in by every intelligent man and woman in

Christendom. And yet our learned professors seem to expect to keep the public mind in darkness on this important subject merely by ridicule.

One in particular, who for twenty-seven years has been held as the champion of America in opposition to it, although he commenced with the promise not to "treat it by ridicule, but by argument," and with the expressed expectation of utterly demolishing it in a single hour, has never to this day been known to devote to the subject a single hour, or even five minutes, in anything but ridicule.

When called before the trustees of the Hospital, in the case already referred to, with facts and arguments sufficient to convince any candid mind of its truth and importance, put in his hands beforehand for the purpose of answering, his attention to them being repeatedly called by direct questions, he evaded every one of them, and spent at least two hours in frivolous ridicule — most of the time in reciting isolated passages from an old homeopathic book, which, in their proper connection, illustrated an important principle, but which, by perversion, were made to show that homeopathists had no more important business than teaching how to cure hiccough and sneezing.

Another doctor tells his patients that homeopathists are not honest; that while they pretend to give only infinitesimal doses, they actually do give the most virulent poisons; and to prove their assertion, recite some terrible cases of death and deformity thus produced.

I once had a patient, of that class who are content

with no one kind of treatment but for a short time, who came to me from an old school physician, and went from me, after a few weeks, to another. The case was a chronic, incurable scrofulous disease, which sometimes assumed one form, and sometimes another.

About the time she came to me, it assumed the form of a white swelling on the knee; while under my care, for perhaps a week, I gave her, for some symptoms which indicated it, arsenicum, of the fourth dilution — dose, perhaps, the ten thousandth part of a grain every night, in all seven of the ten thousandth parts into which the grain was divided, and very imprudently told her what I was giving, without explaining the amount. She told her new doctor the fact that she had been taking arsenic; and he said he then understood the case perfectly. He had seen a great many similar cases, where arsenic had been given in large doses, that showed that while homeopathy pretended to give simple, inoffensive medicine, it was actually dealing in deadly poisons, &c.

The truth is, that the last man to go to, to get true information respecting homeopathy, is an old school physician. I can speak from experience in this matter, for I ridiculed it for years, without understanding a principle or fact upon which it was founded.

If I looked into their books, it was only for the purpose of finding something ridiculous or inconsistent in them. If I saw a plain case of cure from it, I imputed it to some other influence; and that others of the profession are as ignorant of it to-day as I was twenty-five years ago, is shown by the ridiculous and absurd statements from them to which I have referred.

The principles of homeopathy are so simple that the child can understand them, and so consistent that there is no dispute about them among its advocates, as I have elsewhere explained; so that, while old school practice is as much a matter of experiment to-day as it was fifty years ago, — and there is not now a more settled method of treating disease, some giving one thing and some another for the same symptoms and the same disease, and all abandoning their favorite remedies at least once in ten years, — in homeopathy the same remedies are used for the same symptoms to-day as Hahnemann used fifty years ago; and although every year adds to the list of proved remedies, the virtues of those first proved will be acknowledged to the end of time. One thing only is a matter for experiment, and that within certain limits wide enough to satisfy all reasonable minds, is not, as we shall see, a matter of material consequence. The homeopathic dose can only be determined by experiment.

Hahnemann commenced practising homeopathy by giving, according to the law which he discovered, for any particular symptoms of disease, a dose of the medicine which, according to his provings, would produce similar symptoms, of the same size as he had been accustomed to use in his old school practice; but although he effected some wonderful cures, he soon found that in some cases the disease was made worse, and other symptoms induced quite as troublesome as the old ones, and he tried the experiment of giving smaller doses; and finding they did just as well, with less troublesome symptoms, he gradually diminished the dose till it came to be almost infinitesimal.

And finding an influence from medicine too attenuated, as he thought, to be produced by the substance of medicine, he adopted the theory that, by trituration, a kind of spiritual, or, as he called it, a dynamic influence, is imparted from the medicine to the medium in which it was triturated or dissolved and shaken, so that it might be perpetuated without limit; and, getting almost crazed with this idea, he at one time supposed it would grow stronger and stronger by agitation, till he became afraid to carry those dilutions of medicine with him, especially if riding on horseback, lest it might become dangerously strong.

This last idea, however, he afterwards abandoned, but the dynamic idea he never gave up, and it is still adhered to by many of his followers; and there are homeopathic physicians who believe that high attenuations of medicine are more potent than low, and I believe there are in Boston two or three who rarely use medicine of lower dilution than the thirtieth.

Nothing pertaining to homeopathy has been the source of so much ridicule as these high dilutions, and the favorite amusement of old school practitioners is to go into a calculation of the amount of water required to make these dilutions, never making their calculations according to the manner in which the dilutions are actually made, but always misrepresenting the facts, and representing the thirtieth dilution as an impossibility, inasmuch as it would require all the water of Lake Superior to make it: whereas it would require but a single ounce.

Suppose one drop of the tincture of belladonna were put into ten drops of water, and mixed thoroughly by shaking, that would be the first dilution; one drop of the first diluted with ten other drops of water and shaken, would make the second; and so on to the thirtieth; so that the thirtieth may be made by using three hundred drops, which is less than one ounce. Now who shall say that, according to the known laws of divisibility of matter, the last dilution does not contain some atoms of belladonna as well as the first? if not, who shall say in which of these dilutions the ultimate atoms of belladonna ceased to exist?

I know nothing about dynamic influence, and I see no necessity for resorting to any new principle in matter to account for any influence which has been found to be produced by homeopathic medicines.

My idea of dose, and my reasons for it, are these, and you have them at your own valuation, thinking, as I do, very little of theory on any subject, further than theory is deduced from facts.

What the principle is that relieves pain, or assists Nature in the cure of disease, is known only from its effects; but whatever it is, it resides in the ultimate atoms of which the medical drug or plant is composed. And as no divisibility of a drug or any other substance has ever yet been made so as to reduce it to its ultimate atoms, it cannot be asserted of any dilution or trituration ever yet made, if made according to rule, that it cannot retain an atom of its original medicine, I cannot say that it is impossible for a high dilution to produce an effect.

Nor, in view of the influences which I see about me, of matter quite as infinitesimal, can I join in ridiculing the idea as absurd, or even unreasonable. I have elsewhere referred to spora too small to be detected but by a powerful microscope, which are always found floating in the atmosphere that produces intermittent fever, and which are undoubtedly the cause of that terrible disease, which will prostrate the strongest man, and frequently unfits him for business for months, and even causes death.

And yet I have no reason to suppose the thirtieth dilution of arsenic is more attenuated than the dilution of spora in the atmosphere which produced it. And I suppose the evidence is as conclusive that the thirtieth dilution of arsenic has cured intermittent fever, as that the equally attenuated dilution of spora has produced it. If, therefore, I reject the testimony that such an attenuation of medicine will cure a disease, I could not consistently believe the testimony that such an attenuation of spora will produce it.

I have also referred to the fact that an atmosphere impregnated with emanations from ivy, more diluted probably than the thirtieth dilution, — at least the atoms are too small to be detected by a microscope, — will in some persons produce a disease that will shut up their eyes with swelling, and keep them in bed for weeks. Why then should I ridicule the idea that the thirtieth dilution of dogwood — which is known to produce similar symptoms — should cure it?

But the fact that it is possible to cure intermittent fever, or poison, with the thirtieth dilution does not prove that the thirtieth dilution is the best form of medicine to be used in these or any other diseases. Indeed, the inference from the fact connected with the taking of intermittent fever and other diseases from similar dilutions of atoms of the poison which may produce them, prove clearly to my mind that the high dilutions are not as reliable as the low; and this also accords with my own observation in regard to the effects of different dilutions of medicine.

There is certainly an analogy between the effects of homeopathic medicine in curing a disease, and those of infinitely small atoms of poison in inducing disease, as in the cases just referred to. Let us carry out that analogy, and see if we may not get some light on the question of the homeopathic dose.

Let twenty men ride rapidly within twenty feet of ivy, and probably not more than one of this number would be so susceptible to the influences of this poison as to be affected by so slight an influence from it; but let the same twenty men handle the ivy, or have it in the room with them, and perhaps nineteen would be poisoned by it. But the man who took the poison by riding by it would probably be as seriously affected as the others, who could only take it by a stronger influence from it.

This fact we see in other familiar cases. The man who takes small-pox by passing by the house in which it exists, or from a mild case of varioloid, has it just as severely as if he had taken it by coming in contact with one dying from it. He is less likely to take it by passing by the house, or by being in the presence of a mild case; but if he takes it at all, the effect is the same as in the other case.

Insert in the arms of six children matter from the point of a needle so infinitesimal that it requires a microscope to detect it, and into the arms of six other children the same matter from well-charged quills, and many more of the six well vaccinated will take it than of the six that are thus slightly vaccinated; but the pustules of those that do take it from the infinitesimal vaccination will be as perfect and as effectual as the others; but I never vaccinate with a cambric needle, because it is less sure.

And this illustrates my belief and my practice in regard to doses. Very high dilutions, with those who are very susceptible to the influence of the medicine, will produce an effect, just as infinitesimal doses of ivy produced poisonous effects in the individual who was susceptible enough to be influenced by so slight an inoculation; but comparatively few are sufficiently susceptible to be influenced at all by high dilutions, just as few are sufficiently susceptible to ivy to be affected by passing it in the road.

In acute diseases, when an immediate effect is desired, I no more depend on high dilutions than I depend on the matter from the invisible point of a needle in a child exposed to small-pox. And my observation certainly corroborates the theory thus explained.

I have seen some splendid cures with high dilutions in chronic cases, where we could afford to wait; and in such cases they are better than low, because their influence is more permanent; but on the other hand, I am very sure that my high-potency neighbor, who never gives medicine lower than the thirtieth dilution, and claims to be the only pure homeopathist in Boston, makes many more visits, and much larger bills for attendance in the same class of diseases, than the rest of us, who give lower dilutions. His patients are, however, generally satisfied, for he does no harm, and he certainly gives them all the advantages of the expectant treatment, and in chronic cases makes good cures.

But I saw a case of colic which had been treated all night with his high dilutions, being as long as the patient was willing to wait for relief; and she was effectually cured in fifteen minutes by a single dose of medicine of the first dilution.

One shrewd business man, whose wife was induced to try high dilutions, from extravagant promises of cure for some painful pleuritic affection, said, on changing his physician after a long attendance, he thought "high dilutions were well adapted to relieve plethoric pockets, but not to relieve pleurisy."

The true dose of homeopathic medicine, it seems to

me, is that which will soonest and most effectually afford relief, without producing any deleterious effects. The crude drug, even in small doses, does produce injurious effects; I therefore never use it in that form, unless, perhaps, for a single dose. And the first, or perhaps the second dilution, for the same reasons, I give only for a short time; but the third, in acute disease, in which it is never necessary to continue it for a long time, never, in my hands, in a single instance, that I could perceive, has done the slightest harm. And, therefore, as it seems to me to be consummate nonsense to suppose a higher dilution has more curative power than a lower, I never could find a motive to try the high in acute diseases; but in cases where one medicine is to be continued for a long time, the higher seems to retain its influence longer, and, therefore, in chronic diseases, especially in the use of mineral medicines, I use higher. Indeed, I never could conscientiously risk a delay in the cure of a disease by trying experiments with different dilutions.

To use high dilutions in acute diseases seems to me like vaccinating with a cambric needle, and charging for visits till it succeeds, when vaccinating with a hundred times as much matter could in no possible way do harm, while it would be sure to take in the first operation.

Which System is safest for Domestic Practice?

When a child or a friend is sick and in pain, something must be done. Every good impulse of our nature impels us to act, and act immediately. How important, then, to be prepared beforehand to act so as not to do harm, but good. And in view of the facts presented in this and the preceding chapter, I confidently appeal to the common sense of every nurse or mother, and, indeed, of every physician who will lay aside prejudice long enough to give common sense a fair chance, which of the two systems, the heroic or the homeopathic, is safest, and which, in any case of suffering, will be most likely to afford relief?

The choice is between the two, because no mother ever will or can trust to Nature while her child is in pain. She must give some medicine, and the question is, Shall it be crude drugs or homeopathic medicine? Crude medicines always do harm, as we have shown, and this is acknowledged by all sensible physicians who use them, who will tell you they use them "as a choice of evils," — that is, they think the disease will do more harm than the medicine. In this they are mistaken, as has been proved by statistics already given. Why, then, use crude medicine at all?

There are hundreds of families in Boston, who, for fifteen, twenty, and some over thirty years, have not had in their house, or suffered to pass the lips of a single member, a crude or disagreeable medicine for the whole time; and they not only have not been sick more, or suffered longer when sick, than their drug-taking neighbors, but a thousand times less.

And I can testify, in all honesty, that for the last fifteen years, although previously educated to the idea that physics and emetics were necessary in relieving and curing croup, colic, constipation, bilious troubles, &c., I have never seen a case that could not be relieved sooner without than with these or any other crude medicine; and it is more than twenty years since a dose of crude medicine, or anything else offensive to the taste, has been allowed to pass between my lips.

Nothing in this world is more clearly settled, in my mind, than that crude or disagreeable medicines are unnatural means of relieving disease, and, of course, always unnecessary. And next to the hope of heaven, there is nothing that gives me so much comfort, in the prospect of sickness and death, as the assurance that if my senses remain, I shall never, under any circumstances, be tormented with lancets, caustics, cataplasms, emetics, cathartics, or any crude or disgusting drugs.

What any or all of these crude appliances can do of good or evil I ought to understand, having been educated to believe in them, and having practised in that belief faithfully for at least ten years. In the first of my practice I was engaged in a very extensive business with an old heroic disciple of Dr. Rush; and I wish I could forget the mischief we did with antimony, calomel, aloes, calocynth, and the lancet.

One or the other, and sometimes all of which, were tried on a single patient. But the experiment of Louis in the hospitals in Paris, to which I have referred, knocked these abominable notions of practice all out of me, and I soon went over to the belief that all medicines were injurious, and for some ten more years practised on the Hippocratic system of taking care that no harm should be done till Nature should remove the disease.

This was a great improvement over the heroic practice of the preceding ten years, and, excepting the difficulty in satisfying conscience with the deception necessary to keep patients quiet with *placebo* medicines, I was comparatively comfortable, under the impression that I was doing all that could be done.

But at the end of about ten years of expectant practice, a patient, who had suffered for years with chronic bronchitis, and who had thoroughly tried both heroic and expectant treatment, was so indisputably cured by Dr. William Wesselhœft, that I then looked into the merits of homeopathy, and found, instead of the "infinitesimal humbug," which I had previously understood it to be, a beautiful system both in theory and practice, and perfectly consonant with common sense and the common laws of Nature.

And now, having devoted one quarter of my professional life to unmitigated mischief, and one quarter to a harmless but comparatively useless practice, and nearly one quarter more to getting up courage sufficient to face the opposition and persecution of my old friends in the profession, — having, on that account, gone out of the profession for nearly ten years, — I have felt it to be duty for the last ten years, and what remains of life, to do what I could to atone for past offences, not only by practising homeopathy, which I know to be the truth, but also to disseminate its blessed influences in the community in which I live, and, as far as possible, in the world.

The Advantages of Fixed Principles in Medicine.

Aside from the positive advantages of doing right, the peace of mind that comes with a well-grounded faith in the means used for recovery is invaluable in any sickness, not only for the comfort it affords, but as a means of assisting Nature in her indispensable recuperative power. I have seen a stalwart man die for no other apparent reason than that he firmly believed he should die, and had no confidence that any means could save him; and I have seen a confiding, trusting, hoping patient get well against all human probabilities.

In cases of cholera, yellow fever, plague, or any other fatal epidemic, it is noticed that the panic-stricken people who run from place to place to escape it, anxiously inquiring of everybody they meet what they must take, are sure to die, while the calm and confiding nurse, or doctor, or friend who trusts to Providence, and to the means which they believe to be best to preserve and cure them, seldom take the disease, or die if they do take it.

There is nothing so trying in practice as patients who have no confidence in any means of cure — using one day, it may be, the right remedy, but taking at the same time, or soon after, something else that shall entirely counteract all beneficial influences. Such people are always sick, because they never can get well.

Evils of a Vacillating Course of Treatment.

I have seen a shrewd and intelligent business man, not neglectful of the interests of his family, as such men generally are, but remarkably devoted to them, and careful to leave nothing undone that will promote their happiness or prospects, either in this world or in that which is to come, devoting all the time necessary to learn what will be best for them, in health, in the way of schools, amusements, &c., and carefully considering all the advantages or disadvantages of any other proposition pertaining to their welfare; but so perfectly careless respecting what should be done in case of sickness, as not to know whether crude drugs, administered by a regular physician, a quack, or a spiritualist, is best, or whether either are better or not so good as homeopathic medicines.

Accordingly, when sick he goes and takes his children to all by turns, and neither long — going sometimes the whole round of them in a single week. The result is — it must be — that all that is done for them is lost, and worse than lost, for one doctor not only interferes with and counteracts what the other does, but also interferes with Nature's efforts, and the chances of recovery are vastly less than if nothing at all was done.

If he saw a merchant behaving as ridiculously in his trades and investments, buying a cargo of goods, and getting them on board his vessel, and then changing his mind, and selling them at a sacrifice, and buying another kind to take their place; sending vessels to Cuba with warming-pans, and then to Greenland with ice, he would call him a fool, and would know that he would soon become bankrupt.

But is it less absurd, or less sure to produce bankruptcy in health, to treat a constitutional disease with local effects — at one time with medicines to drive it out of the system, and at another with local remedies to drive it back again into the blood? If he would take a sixteenth part of the time to inquire and find out which is right and which is wrong in medical practice, that he takes to investigate the security of a single investment, he would never do such wrongs to himself and his children.

And what a difference, in peace of mind in sickness, between a man who knows the right and steadily pursues it, turning neither to the right or left, nor regarding the importunities of his ignorant and importunate neighbors, and the man who, not knowing what is right, is "driven about by every wind of doctrine," — distracted by finding that to please one neighbor he has been doing his child harm, and then to please another has been doing equal harm in another direction.

HOW TO SELECT MEDICINES IN CASE OF SICKNESS.

THE manner in which the medical virtues of drugs and plants are ascertained, I have elsewhere partly explained, but not fully. A number of persons of different ages, temperaments, sexes, &c., at stated times, each take a given dose of medicine, — generally without knowing what is taken, — each keeping a record by himself of any peculiar sickness, pains, or other symptoms or changes that occur in a given time, and noting the order of their occurrence.

If the medicine has any active properties, it will be found, on comparing notes, that some of the effects will be the same on nearly all who tried the experiment; other effects will be the same on only part, and perhaps a small part, of those who took it; and some, perhaps, who are not susceptible to the influence of that particular medicine, are not affected at all.

Some will have very severe pains or other symptoms, and others will have the same kind of pains in the same parts of the system, but less severe, and perhaps very slight. It will be found, also, that those of the same sex will have peculiar effects, differing from those of the other sex; that those of the same complexion and temperament will have similar effects, differing from the effects on those of a different complexion or temperament.

Now, in case of the occurrence of similar pains or symptoms, in the same part of the body, as those which were produced by the medicine tested in most of the individuals who tested it, a little, no matter how little, within reasonable limits, will certainly relieve those pains or symptoms, unless the patient happens to be an exception, like the exceptions referred to, in which that particular medicine has no influence; and these exceptions are as rare as the exceptions to its influence found in testing it.

If the symptoms are of the class of which only a few were affected in the provings, then the probabilities of relief are less, and dependent on the fact whether they belong to the same sex or temperament as those affected by the provings. And this shows how much study and how much judgment are required to practice homeopathy, having three or four hundred medicines to select from, and new ones are being proved every day.

Homeopathy, therefore, instead of being that ridiculous humbug which it is represented to be, is not only the most important and most interesting of the sciences, but requires the most judgment and the most study to apply it practically to the varied and varying phases of disease as they come before us, and as a study it is absolutely inexhaustible. Nevertheless, the colds, inflammations, fevers, bilious troubles, bowel and stomach difficulties, which are the principal sources of the sufferings in families, produce symptoms which are almost all produced by a few well-proved medicines — at least as many of them as most families are willing to contend with, without medical advice.

Our books on domestic medicines are mostly too large and too complicated, and in case of sickness it requires too much study to select a remedy adapted to the case. They devote a large part of the book to describing diseases, calling them by name, which, being alike in their essential characteristics, and requiring the same remedies, might as well all be described together in one single paragraph, or, at least, in very few paragraphs.

For example: in "Family Homeopathy," by Ellis, you will find more than three hundred pages devoted to the description of different kinds of fevers and inflammations, as bilious fever, scarlet fever, colds in the head, pleurisy, pericarditis, hepatitis, pneumonia, &c. — to each of which is given a repetition of the same prescriptions, as the first thing to be done, viz.: give aconite, and, if the pain and soreness are local, use a compress with cold water, covered with dry flannel.

If a mother wishes to find out what first to do for her child, when hot, and feverish, or sore in a particular place, and it hurts to touch it or to move, why need she be compelled to read for two hours, to find out whether the disease is pleurisy, or pericarditis, or hepatitis, before giving it relief, when, after all her research, and whatever conclusions she comes to on that point, the remedy is the same? Why not apply the compress and give the aconite at once, and hunt up the name afterwards, if it must be had?

In doubtful and obstinate cases, a physician may derive much advantage from knowing the particular organ affected, in order more scientifically to apply his remedies, some medicines being adapted to one organ and some another; but why should a mother bother herself with such inquiries, especially if she must leave her child to suffer while going into this useless inquiry?

When a child is taken with fever or pain, and the mother sees it suffering, she will do something for it, right or wrong, and study up the case when more at leisure. She wants to know what to do for such symptoms; and I propose to devote a few pages to the symptoms to which, in our wrong mode of living, which I have elsewhere explained, we are all liable, and to the remedies which Nature has provided for the relief of those symptoms.

My purpose is not to induce people to dispense with the services of a physician, for I will not presume that intelligent mothers will be foolhardy enough to take the responsibility of carrying a precious child, without advice, through a dangerous fit of sickness. It is the very ignorant only who dare do that, if good advice can be had; for those who consider how little he knows of the laws of life, and the laws of disease, who devotes his life to the study of them, must feel that she must know much less whose thoughts and time are devoted to other things.

But I do think that a consideration of the virtues of a few of the common remedies, and the leading symptoms they are adapted to relieve, will enable any intelligent mother to relieve nine out of ten of the pains and ills to which her children are subject, and that without ever resorting to a crude and disgusting article of medicine, or allowing her children to suffer a single pain for the want of it.

It will, in the gravest cases, at least enable her to afford some relief, without danger of doing harm, till medical advice can be obtained. For those who live far away from any good physician, some good book on domestic practice, describing more particularly diseases and their remedies, is desirable.

And perhaps there is no one yet published combining more valuable instruction than that to which I have referred by Dr. Ellis; but it has the defects to which I have referred. And I venture the assertion, that although it is as faultless in this respect as any treatise on domestic remedies yet published, yet, in the way I have suggested, a writer capable of condensing ideas might bring these four hundred pages into less than one hundred, retaining every important idea, and enabling the reader to find out in fifteen minutes all that from this could be extracted in an hour. And it has another important defect. Although an edition has been published this very year (1868), it ignores every medicine, with perhaps one exception, that has been proved within the last twenty years. And yet, beyond a few of the forty-eight remedies on which he depends, there are not any on which I with more confidence and satisfaction depend than on some that I can select from Hale's New Remedies.

For a book containing the improvements suggested above I have long seen the necessity, and have sometimes threatened to try to supply the deficiency; but hitherto have found no time. Meantime I think I can condense into a very limited space all that any family needs to know who depends on a physician for grave and dangerous diseases, and who only desire to know what to do first in severe cases till advice can be had, and what to continue to do in cases requiring no medical advice.

What to do first in Case of Sickness.

How to treat Inflammations.

In all cases occurring in cold weather give aconite the first thing, and if there be severe local pain or soreness, apply to the place of pain or soreness, or to the nearest point possible, a compress larger or smaller, according to the size of the part to which the pain is referred, consisting of four or five thicknesses of a folded napkin, or other linen or cotton cloth, wrung out of cold water, and two or three thicknesses of dry flannel over it. Let this medicine be taken, and this wet cloth be changed in all except extraordinary cases at first once an hour, and in very severe sufferings every fifteen minutes. This in all cases will be safe practice long enough to get advice, or to develop some other symptoms requiring some other remedy.

How to treat Croup.

In case of severe croup, or affection of the organs of voice, after repeating the cold application and the aconite two or three times every fifteen minutes, as before advised, give, in alternation with aconite, hepar sulphur; at first every fifteen minutes, and less and less often as the symptoms subside, changing the compress as often as the medicine is given.

How to treat Pleurisy or other similar Diseases.

In case of pleurisy, or any sharp, severe pains anywhere, alternate bryonia with aconite, more or less often according to the severity of the pain, changing the compress, and diminishing the frequency of medicine, as in the case of croup.

How to treat Swelled Tonsils.

In case of inflammation of the throat, with red swelling of the tonsils, alternate belladonna with aconite, changing the compress on the throat, and using the medicines as directed in the foregoing cases.

How to treat Diphtheria.

In case of swelled tonsils, with white specks or a buff-colored coating on them, use phytolacca with aconite, as in the foregoing cases, leaving off the compress, and giving up the aconite for baptisia as soon as there is coldness of the skin, using warm dry flannel instead of the wet bandage, and alternating the medicines every hour.

How to treat Colds.

If the inflammation settles, as in a cold, in the nasal passages, eyes or ears, or back of the throat, alternate with aconite, for the first day, æsculus hippocastanum, and the next day hydrastes, alternating the two last named medicines instead of the aconite, two or three times each in the twenty-four hours.

How to treat Coughs.

If cough or soreness of the lungs occurs, use at first sticta in alternation with aconite, and when it becomes loose, bryonia; and if these fail, or if the cough continues dry after a few days, gelseminum and tart. antimony.

How to treat Inflammation of the Bladder.

If the inflammation settles in the bladder, and painful or too frequent micturition is the consequence, alternate the aconite with cantharides, using the compress as before, for the first twenty-four hours; afterwards alternate gelseminum and hydrastes.

How to treat Rheumatism.

If the inflammation is rheumatic, and the muscles or joints are sore, and it hurts to move them, alternate bryonia with aconite for forty-eight hours, if necessary, and if no relief is experienced, change the medicines, and alternate gelseminum with caulophylum for one day, and the next day substitute phytolacca for caulophylum.

When to stop taking Medicine.

In all these cases, and all other cases, stop the medicine as soon as the symptoms are relieved.

How to treat Diseases in warm Weather.

In warm weather, and in warm climates, another and different class of diseases are most prevalent. While in winter the exciting cause of disease is generally catching cold, in warm weather the exciting cause is generally indigestion, the principal predisposing cause being the same in both cases — too much carbonaceous food, which tends to produce extra heat and extra work for all the organs, rendering them more susceptible to disease.

In winter, the inflammations and diseases are greatly under the influence of aconite. In summer, they are more influenced by nux vomica than any other one article; at least all the colics, and cramps, and flatulence, and diarrhœas, which come from undigested food, are relieved, in grown persons of full habits or dark complexions, by nux; but in children these symptoms are best relieved by chamomilla, and in delicate females more perhaps by pulsatilla.

How to treat Cramps and Colics.

If a severe pain is felt in the stomach or bowels, which is produced by undigested food, or from a constipated habit, or from an unknown cause, nux vomica is the remedy most likely to afford relief; and if it be accompanied with fever and heat in the parts affected, use the cold compress and aconite with the nux, in alternations; but if the patient be cold, make warm applications instead of the cold compress, and use veratrum instead of aconite. If nux fails, colocynth is to be used instead.

How to treat Diarrhœa.

If diarrhœa comes on in consequence of undigested food, accompanied with pain, nux will relieve the pain while Nature removes the cause. If the diarrhœa is without pain, and colorless, veratrum is the remedy; if it be bilious, podophylon; and if accompanied by sickness, ipecac or arsenicum, with flour porridge, or other food containing no waste.

How to treat Dysentery.

If there be forcing pain in the lower part of the bowels, and bloody or slimy discharges, corrosive mercury, with aconite, at first, afterwards gelseminum and colocynth, and if they fail, hippocastanum or collinsonia.

How to treat Constipation.

If habitually constipated, collinsonium every night, with food containing waste,* for one week, and hydrastes in the same way for the next, till the bowels will act without these remedies; but never take cathartic medicine, or aperient pills or powders, which, though for the day give relief, yet always increase the difficulty; but if absolutely necessary, take an enema instead.

* See Philosophy of Eating, page 121.

Cathartics not necessary.

Cathartics or emetics are never necessary to assist in removing pain or disease; and for twenty years I have never seen a case of suffering from colics, cramps, stoppage, or bilious obstructions, that could not be relieved sooner without than with either cathartics or emetics.

Even if the pain be occasioned by the presence of a foreign substance, as cherry stones, or other indigestible substances, it is much sooner relieved by nux, colocynth, or belladonna, which relaxes the spasm that causes the pain by contracting the intestine and holding on to the offending substance, and lets it pass on; whereas cathartic medicines often prolong and intensify the suffering by increasing the irritation and the spasm. Thus also, what is called a stoppage, which is a spasmodic contraction of the intestine, caused by some irritating substance, is much sooner relieved without than with cathartic medicine. This I affirm confidently, having tried both methods of cure scores if not hundreds of times.

Exceptional Cases in which Cathartics are necessary.

The only contingency in which for twenty years I have found a cathartic necessary, is one in which there is imbedded in the folds of the intestines some foreign substance, which Nature is unable to remove, as in the following instance: A gentleman who, conceiving the idea that the seeds of barberry were good for dyspepsia, had eaten them daily for three or four years, and had swallowed in all perhaps two or three hundred pounds, suffering all the time with colics, which were occasionally terribly severe.

Suspecting the cause of the suffering, — indeed, being able to feel the balls of accumulated seeds through the parietes of the abdomen, — he was put upon a course of lubricating, oily cathartics, with the result of obtaining some pounds of these impacted balls of barberry seeds, and of curing him at the same time of the absurd idea of treating dyspepsia with any such crude and irritating materials.

How to cure Neuralgia.

Neuralgia, as its name indicates, is pain of the nerves, and it is distinguished from pain induced by rheumatism, or other inflammations, by this distinction: Pain from rheumatism or other inflammations is always accompanied with soreness, and increase of suffering on motion; while in neuralgia there is no increase of pain by motion, and very little, if any, soreness.

Neuralgia seems to be caused, as I have before explained, by too much heating food, and is indeed a kind of inflammation; but the nerves affected are generally covered over with muscle and adipose matter, which protect them from the effects of pressure, and not being directly concerned, as the muscles are in the motion of the part, are not affected in the same way; but when neuralgia is brought on by cold, the same means are adopted to relieve it as other inflammations — aconite and a cold compress.

But there are forms of neuralgia connected with the digestive organs, and these will be relieved by the same remedies that relieve pain in the bowels, to which I have referred. At any rate, excepting in cases occurring from catching cold, nux, colocynth, and veratrum, in the order in which I place them, are effectual in relieving neuralgic pains; and in case of great prostration and debility, gelseminum alternated with veratrum, or with arsenicum, or with phytolacca; and these are all the remedies I should dare recommend without getting advice.

How to treat Headaches.

Headaches are produced by one of three causes — by constipation or indigestion; by over-heated blood; and by neuralgia. These may all be cured and prevented by appropriate means, and by living according to the laws of life, as explained in the Philosophy of Eating. Of this I speak confidently, having seen many examples of cure in each class of headaches, in the young and in the old, and having seen no case, however severe, that could not be relieved by medicine, and prevented by appropriate diet.

One lady of seventy, who all her lifetime had been subject to sick headaches, and her mother before her, and who for some years, up to the last five years, had been confined to her bed with them nearly one quarter of the time, sometimes for three or four weeks at a time, for the last five years is only troubled when she breaks her rules of diet, and then is relieved in a few hours by medicines which she keeps by her. Her case is only extraordinary in its severity and in the length of time it had been endured.

The importance of living philosophically in cases of headache from over-heated blood, has been impressed on me by my own experience, having been subject to them from my earliest recollection till the age of fifty, and having frequently been obliged to remain in bed for a whole day in excruciating suffering; and now living as nearly as possible according to the laws of life, I have not for some years felt a twinge of headache that I remember; and for fourteen years have been exempt except as a direct penalty for some indulgence in extra carbonaceous food.

In such cases it would seem to be but justice that we should suffer without the means of relief, till we had paid the full penalty for our transgressions, and by our sufferings should be compelled to obey the laws of life. But if our heavenly Father, in his infinite mercy, has furnished us the means of relieving even the sufferings caused directly by our transgressions, it is certainly right that we should avail ourselves of them; and I therefore will explain the means of relief in the different forms of headache, — not with a view to induce any one not acquainted with the laws of disease, and the various considerations which vary the treatment so that no two chronic cases are to be treated alike, to attempt to cure themselves of chronic or long-standing headache of either kind. This can be done only by a homeopathic physician of good judgment and skill. But temporary relief in most cases can be obtained by studying the following suggestions: —

How to relieve Headache induced by Indigestion.

That which will relieve indigestion will relieve the pains induced by it; and accordingly we find that headaches, when accompanied with constipation, will be relieved by collinsonia or hydrastes, and if connected with foul tongue, pains in the stomach and bowels, or oppression from flatulence, nux will afford relief in constitutions to which nux is adapted by temperament, &c.; otherwise, pulsatilla or hydrastes. If the right remedy be found, in those who are subject to attacks of headache it will afford relief very soon, often by a single dose if taken at first; but at most two or three doses, taken every hour, will be all that is required in the worst cases.

I know very many cases of persons subject to attacks of sick headache, which comes from indigestion, who had previously been obliged to spend the whole day in bed, who, by taking a single dose, or at most, two doses of nux, when the first symptoms are felt, soon forget their headache, and keep about their business as usual; and so reliable are its effects, that no time has been lost for months or years, whereas, before resorting to this means of relief, hours were lost every month from it. Other articles are best adapted to other cases, of which any good homeopathic physician can judge; and I have come firmly to believe there is no such thing as incurable headache from indigestion.

How to cure Headache induced by over-heated Blood.

Here, too, we must apply common sense to general principles. That which will cure inflammations which are induced by over-heated blood will cure headaches from the same cause; accordingly, when headache is accompanied with flushed face, and a sense of pressure, and fulness and throbbing of the blood vessels, aconite always gives relief. And cold water applied directly to the head, or, what is more philosophical and more effectual, applied to the throat, so as to cool the blood of the arteries as it passes very near the surface, — and this last is an important suggestion, not only in common congestive headaches but in all headaches accompanied with fever, — a cold compress to the throat affords much more effectual relief than if applied directly to the head; but there is no harm, in severe cases, in making both appliances.

How to treat Nervous Headaches.

Headaches usually denominated nervous are generally neuralgic, and are to be treated upon the same principles and with the same remedies as neuralgia, whether induced by cold or induced by and connected with derangement of the digestive organs; and therefore no distinctive treatment can be given, except such as has been referred to under neuralgia, headaches from indigestion, and from over-heated blood. For doubtful cases it is safest to consult a physician.

HOMEOPATHIC MEDICINES.

OUR ailments, in a temperate climate, in which we have a cold and a warm season, may be comprised in the foregoing list; and, as far as they can be supposed to be understood by intelligent mothers, can be as well treated by the list of about twenty remedies as by the three or four hundred that have been tested: for to those who do not make medicine a professional study, the larger the number to select from, the more doubt as to which is the right one. And a small list of remedies, by considering the leading and characteristic symptoms which each is adapted to cure, can be varied to suit different symptoms as they come up. To assist in making such variation in practice, I will give the leading peculiarities of each of the twenty medicines referred to, as they have been developed by provings, and as these provings have been corroborated by thousands of cases in which they have been used.

First, however, let me refer to an interesting fact, showing the same Providential care in adapting medicines to each particular climate as that, to which I have elsewhere referred, in adapting food to the wants of each climate. As in cold climates, where more heat is required, more oil and starch are furnished in the meats and the grains, producing, with other heating materials, more inflammations and inflammatory fevers than less heating food, so in the same climate are furnished the medical plants best adapted to cure these inflammations. Aconite, bryonia, belladonna, &c., the articles on which we mostly depend for the cure of these diseases, grow in northern regions only; while nux vomica, colocynth, and gelseminum, which are adapted to relieve the diseases induced in warm climates and warm weather, grow only in warm climates.

Aconite is found in the mountainous regions of the north of Europe and America; bryonia, also, in Northern Europe; and belladonna is a common weed in the Northern American States. Gelseminum, which is adapted to the fevers of warm weather, as aconite is to cold, grows only in the Southern States, and nux and colocynth only in India. And when the *materia medica* is more nearly perfected (we have not yet had time to perfect it since we found the key by which to unlock Nature's medical treasures), we shall probably find that every climate in which man can live is furnished with its own remedies, sufficient to cure all the diseases and relieve all the pains to which its inhabitants are subject.

The following is a list of the remedies to which I have referred, and the leading symptoms which each is adapted to relieve. It will be seen that, while many of the remedies have symptoms in common with others, every one has some symptoms peculiar to itself; and this is found to be true with regard to every article of medicine that has yet been proved.

Aconite

Produces, and therefore will cure, acute local inflammations; fevers of an inflammatory character; congestion, or sense of fulness of the lungs, or head, or any other organ; neuralgia or rheumatism, or any other sharp pains, with or without swelling; thirst, and flushed face, with dry skin; sleeplessness and restlessness; dryness of the mouth and tongue; loss of appetite, and sense of oppression and lassitude, with a feeling of general repletion and uneasiness.

Arsenicum.

Extreme weakness and debility; emaciation; sinking of the strength; coldness of the feet and hands; and the pains, and fevers, and restless sleeplessness which accompanies the foregoing symptoms. Also many diseases of the skin; but these can only be judiciously prescribed for by an experienced physician.

Belladonna.

Startings of the limbs; convulsions; loss of consciousness; red swellings of the tonsils; redness of the skin, and scarlet eruptions; boring and stinging of the skin; congestion or inflammation of the eyes, and pain in the eyeballs or back of the eyes; delirium; dizziness; confusion of mind; headache over the eyes, and throbbing pain in the temples; colic pains; bright red tongue, and burning in the mouth and throat.

Baptisia.

Sense of prostration of the whole system — soreness of the flesh on pressure; incapable of making exertions; pains are increased by motion and relieved by rest; hands, arms, and legs tremulous; bloated, distended feeling about the eyes; burning heat of the face; profuse flow of saliva; throat feels swollen, but is not; tickling in the throat provoking cough; sense of tightness about the chest; dull, heavy pains in the back; aching of the limbs, with sense of weariness.

Bryonia.

Sharp pains in the side, aggravated by breathing; stiffness, and pain, and swelling in the joints; trembling of the limbs when at rest; pains aggravated by motion or contact, relieved by rest; jarring headache, as if the brain were loose, aggravated by stooping; white coating on the tongue; pressure in the stomach after eating; cough, with soreness of the chest, either dry or loose; painful stiffness of the nape of the neck; pains in the back and limbs, with soreness and stiffness.

Cantharides.

This medicine has a specific effect on the urinary organs, as in old school practice I had frequent proof. Blisters applied to any part of the body frequently produce irritation of these organs, with painful micturition. For all such irritations this medicine will afford relief in homeopathic doses.

Chamomilla.

A medicine particularly adapted to infants and small children, for irritability, restlessness, constant crying, and the thousand and one little ills that come with the process of teething. Given occasionally it has great influence, but given too frequently it loses its influence.

Colocynth.

For all colics, cramps, griping pains, especially of the stomach and bowels.

Collinsonia.

Constipation, with the diseases produced by it, and all painful diseases of the bowels and urinary organs.

Gelseminum.

This medicine takes the place of aconite, in the cure of fevers, inflammations, pains, and nervous symptoms, with this distinctive difference: aconite is adapted to active diseases of cold weather, gelseminum to the less active diseases of warm weather. It is also very useful in nervous prostration and partial paralysis, especially for those symptoms occurring with diphtheria.

Hepar Sulphur.

Croupy affections, or hoarseness and sense of suffocation; itching diseases of the skin, with pimples or sores; suppurating wounds, which heal tardily, with unhealthy acrid discharges.

Hydrastes.

Inflammations of the mucous membrane of the nose, eyes, mouth, throat, or lower organs; aphthous or cankery spots in the mouth, especially of children; weakness of stomach, and incipient indigestion; mucous discharges from any part of the mucous membrane.

Hippocastanum.

Cold in the head, with stupefying pain in the head, and watery discharges from nose and eyes; pains in the bowels, very low; and all painful diseases of the lower abdominal organs, with pain in the back; constipation and piles.

Ipecacuanha.

Sickness at stomach, and vomiting, with dizziness; asthmatic breathing, and wheezing cough; bleeding from the lungs, stomach, or bowels; yellowness of the skin.

Mercurius Corrosivus.

Ulcerated condition of mouth and throat; swelling and tenderness of the gums; profuse salivation, or watery discharge from the glands of the mouth; canker sores; bloody discharges with pain, as in dysentery.

Nux Vomica.

Next to aconite, there is no medicine yet proved that relieves so great a variety of distressing symptoms as nux vomica. Its influence seems to be mainly through the brain and nervous system; and in different forms and applications, which the physician only can understand, it relieves symptoms of apparently opposite character, as violent spasms and paralysis. For domestic use it would be serviceable in indigestion, colics, croup, and neuralgia; but for other diseases, other remedies are more reliable, for non-professional practitioners.

Phytolacca.

This medicine has great influence on the glandular system, and especially on the breasts. It is useful in all swellings of the glands of any part of the system. In large doses, often repeated, it carries off the flesh by absorption; in small doses it tends to restore lost flesh. It is valuable in diphtheria, and in dull white or gray swelling of the mouth or throat. And within the last few years, since scarlet fever is accompanied with this diphtherious kind of inflammation, phytolacca, to a great extent, takes the place of belladonna in the treatment of it.

Podophylon.

Yellowness of the skin and eyes, indicating obstructions in the liver; sleepiness and tired feeling, with dizziness and headache; offensive breath, and copious flow of saliva; nausea and throbbing at the stomach; pains in the region of the liver; diarrhœa, and forcing pains.

Pulsatilla.

Peculiarly adapted to the ailments and pains to which the female constitution is subject; and to the hysterical and nervous irregularities, as well as the painful obstructions, to which that sex alone is subject.

Sticta Pulmonaria.

Pains in the bones; darting pains in the arms and legs, with sense of fulness about the nose, indicating an approaching cold; burning of the eyes and eyelids, with sharp, darting pains about the head; cough, with soreness of lungs, tickling in the throat, and raising specks of blood.

Tartarized Antimony.

Cough, with great prostration, difficulty of breathing, constriction of the chest, expectoration of bloody matter; excessive vomiting, with great exhaustion, and cramps of the stomach.

Veratrum.

Veratrum is useful in diseases of weakness and depression, with cold feet and hands; but its principal use in domestic practice is for painless, watery diarrhœa of children in summer.

Errors in the Use of Medicines.

In using homeopathic medicines, two or three errors are to be guarded against. It is a common and natural feeling that if a certain amount of medicine is expected to cure a disease in a given time, say twenty-four hours, twice the amount will cure it in twelve hours; and medicine is given too often, if not in too large doses. Beyond the amount necessary to effect the cure, all medicine is injurious, and often produces and increases unpleasant symptoms. Another error consists in continuing medicine too long. As a rule, it should be given less and less often as the symptoms subside, and be stopped when they are removed, otherwise new symptoms are induced or old ones renewed. With these precautions, the cure of any disease may be hastened, without any possible harm, by homeopathic medicine. If in doubt on this point, take two children with colds alike, and give to one medicine as directed, and trust the other to Nature, with the same diet and care in other respects, and the one that takes the medicine will require less than half the time to get well as the other.

WHAT IS SUN-STROKE?

THE alarming number of deaths reported as from sun-stroke at every heated period makes it important to understand the cause of these deaths and the means of preventing them. To explain it intelligibly, we must revert to that beautiful chemico-vital principle explained in Philosophy of Eating, pages 178 to 183, by which the temperature of the body, in all external temperatures, and all degrees of exercise; in sickness and health, is kept at nearly the same point, seldom varying more than one or two degrees from 98, and never having been known to vary only from 96.5 to 102, this being the utmost range of variation in which life can be sustained. This regulation of temperature is effected by the evaporation of perspiration from the surface of the body, according to the law of Nature, instituted probably for the very purpose, that evaporation produces cold. If a bottle of wine, or any other liquid, be covered with a wet cloth, and placed in a draught of air, the drying of the cloth abstracts the heat from the liquid, and thus under the equator can be had drinks almost as cool as ice-water. This effect we also experience in sitting in a draught of air, in the cold we catch. By the same process, by a vital power which cannot be explained, a similar evaporation is constantly kept up on the surface of the body, to carry off the surplus heat that is generated within. If the weather is cold, and we keep still so as not to generate much heat, no surplus being generated, and no evaporation necessary, the pores of the skin are closed, and no moisture being on the surface, no evaporation takes place; but if the weather be warm, and we have violent exercise to generate heat rapidly, the pores are open, and perspiration oozes through them to just the extent necessary to abstract the extra heat as it is generated. The amount of drink required to supply this evaporation is of course proportionate to the heat and the exercise, and the sense of thirst indicates what is needed.

If this natural process is not interfered with, and the wants of Nature are supplied, we can endure almost any amount of external heat, even that sufficient to cook meat, as in the examples given in Philosophy of Eating, page 181, the evaporation in these cases carrying off the heat to this astonishing degree; but if the pores of the skin were obstructed or closed in such cases, death would ensue immediately; or if the supply of perspiration were deficient, or the vital power exhausted, so that the perspiration could not be kept up, the internal temperature rising only three or four degrees above 98, death ensues immediately.

Now in cases of death from sun-stroke, one of four things must be the immediate cause of it: — the pores of the skin are closed, so as to stop perspiration; or the supply of drink is not sufficient to support the requisite perspiration; or the vital powers are exhausted, so as not to be able to carry on the process of perspiration to the extent necessary to keep down the internal temperature; or the temperature is suddenly brought below 96° by cold drinks. In either of these contingencies, the internal temperature rises to 102° or 104°, or sinks below 96°, and we are gone at once. Facts obtained from the intelligent agent of the Metropolitan Horse Railroad Company corroborate the theory explained above. Formerly, in hot seasons, they lost every year very many horses, all dying suddenly, and with similar premonitory symptoms. The first noticeable change was, that they stopped sweating; then soon, if kept at work, they would falter, and fall down and die. These sudden deaths were sometimes induced by drinking cold water, with the same results, unless the heat could be soon raised again, by warm drinks, &c. Seeing this effect of water, and not realizing that it was the cold and not the water that produced this fatal effect, the horses were allowed but little water; and this increased the danger. They have lately changed their treatment, giving them all the water they will drink, of the temperature of the air at the time; and during the last uncommonly hot season, in which hundreds of horses and men have died under similar circumstances, they have not, of their eight hundred horses, lost a single one. When a tired horse, in a hot day, is seen to stop sweating, they take him out of the harness, sponge the skin with water not too cold, cover him with a blanket, and give him warm water, — that is, water that has stood for some time in the open air, — and he always recovers; and when the weather is very hot, they drive very slowly, so as not to heat their blood.

Here, then, we have a clew to the cause, as before described, and an intimation of the means of preventing and curing this fatal malady.

I have also obtained some facts, which tend to the same conclusions, from the habits of firemen in furnaces, glass-houses, and steamboats. From the late surgeon of the Pacific steamships I learn that the firemen work over the fire in an atmosphere, on an average, of forty degrees higher than the temperature of the blood. To keep the heat of the blood down to the point at which life can be sustained, under such circumstances, requires an amount of perspiration and an amount of drink perfectly enormous. To sustain this exhausting process they formerly used switchel, — molasses and water, — sometimes with a little vinegar. Under the use of that drink they were subject to distressing colics, or cramps, and not knowing what produced them, the surgeon introduced, instead of the switchel, water in which had been stirred barley, corn or oatmeal; and from that time they endured the heat much better, and never afterwards had the cramps or colics. I learn, also, that in most of the iron and glass making establishments in Europe where firemen are thus exposed, they drink as much as they please of oatmeal or barley water, prepared as before suggested, and they endure their exhausting labor in the enjoyment of excellent health.

In other similar establishments they drink freely of pure water, of the temperature of the atmosphere; but wherever they use, in the enormous quantities necessary, beer or switchel, or any other drinks containing carbonaceous or heating principles, they are subject to pains and other difficulties.

Means of preventing and curing Sun-stroke.

From the foregoing suggestions, it is safe to infer that, as a preventive of the disease called sun-stroke, — although the sun has evidently nothing to do with it directly, — under any exhausting exercise, in any temperature, a free use of pure water at the temperature of the atmosphere, or water in which is infused the life and strength-giving elements found in the meal of all unbolted grains, avoiding any very cold drinks, should be indulged in. And in case of attack, warm and stimulating drinks, with sponging and gentle friction of the skin, and perfect rest of the muscles, as the best means of recovery.

Seeing the evil effects of cold water, — which are only worse than other drinks because more of it is usually taken, — and supposing the evil to come from the water and not from the cold, men exposed to excessive heat are apt to take too little liquids to sustain the perspiration, and that causes the very evil which they wish to avoid. The cold only is to be avoided, as it is that which produces a chill or shock to the vital organs, in which the stomach comes in contact, suddenly stopping the vital action, and reducing the temperature of the blood below the point at which life can be sustained.

The Predisposing Causes of Sun-stroke.

I find, on inquiry, that the horses which fall down and die in hot days are never lean and shabby ones, but always the fattest; and the men who die of sun-stroke are those who live on carbonaceous and stimulating food, generally also heating their blood with alcoholic stimulants, and have not enough of the nitrogenous or phosphatic elements to give power to sustain any exhausting influence. In such men molasses and water only increase the heat of the blood, without giving recuperative power to sustain it; but the water diffused in meal takes up only nitrogenous and phosphatic elements, the starch not being soluble in cold water, and from it is obtained power to sustain the exhausting influence of the perspiration; and where this influence is long continued, such drink must be of essential service.

Fat horses and fat men suffer more than lean ones, because the adipose covering, being a non-conductor, retains the heat, and renders the perspiration less effectual. This can be understood by reference to the process of cooling drinks by evaporation, as in the cases referred to. If, instead of applying the wet cloth directly to the bottle of drink, it were first enveloped in flannel, with the wet cloth over that, the effect of evaporation would be greatly diminished. From this we may infer that fat men should keep still in hot weather.

GOUT: ITS CAUSE AND CURE.

In the chapters on general inflammations and neuralgia, we have seen that the predisposing cause of inflammations and pains is carbonaceous food, heating, as it does, the blood, the internal organs, and the nerves, as the fire of a steamboat heats the combustible materials around the boiler, and renders them more susceptible to ignition. This illustration is particularly applicable to the gout, which is eminently painful and inflammatory; and it is corroborated by the fact that subjects for the gout are generally fat, and live *high*, which, according to the English and American acceptation of that term, means that their food is greatly composed of butter, fat, starch, and sugar, in which, as we have seen in Philosophy of Eating, page 18, are only the heat-producing elements, without either strength-giving principles for the muscles, or food for the brain and nerves. But there are some peculiarities of the gout which distinguish it from all other inflammatory diseases.

One exciting cause of gout is violent, exciting, or long-continued mental action — an exciting cause of no other inflammatory disease; at least the effects are peculiar to gout, and the disease is accompanied with peculiar irritability of mind, irascibility of temper, and frequently with deposits of certain effete matter as it passes from the system. Let us see if these peculiarities are not susceptible of explanation.

What physical effect on the system is produced by violent, exciting, or long-continued mental action, such as induces gout?

In Philosophy of Eating, page 87, it is shown that one twelfth of the solid matter of the brain is phosphorus, which is combined with other mineral principles, the most important of which is soda; and that the amount of phosphorus varies in different brains according to mental capacity, children and idiots having less than half as much as men of common intellects.

It is also shown that this phosphorus is used up in thinking, and in any mental exercise, and thrown from the system as effete matter, just as nitrogen is used up and thrown off in working the muscles — clergymen excreting more phosphorus on Monday than any other day of the week, and lawyers excreting more after court days than at any other time.

The Want of Phosphorus the Cause of Gout.

Assuming, then, that the want of phosphorus in the system is the cause of the characteristic symptoms which distinguish gout from other inflammatory diseases, we have a rational explanation of all their phenomena, and a theory of prevention and cure, corroborated by the experience and observation of those who are best acquainted with the disease.

Phosphorus not only promotes the action of the brain, and produces mental activity and power, but it promotes the action of the muscles, and is the source of all nervous or vital power and physical health and activity. This is seen in the examples given in Philosophy of Eating, in which it is proved, by analysis, that the most active animals, birds, or fishes have most phosphorus in the composition of their flesh, and require most phosphatic food to sustain their activity. This principle is also fully explained in the first chapter of this book, on Food for Thinking Men.

I have also explained, in another chapter, the well-known fact that nursing and expectant mothers who live on carbonaceous food suffer from excruciating neuralgia, toothache, &c., because, not taking phosphorus enough in food to keep the nerves of the mother and child both in a healthy condition, Nature favors the child at the expense of the mother.

And here we have a hint of the cause of the excruciating pain accompanying gout, and the reason why not only gouty people, but all other fat people who eat too much carbonaceous food, suffer toothache and all other painful diseases more severely than those who live on natural food.

The Rationale of the Gout, and its Treatment.

Gouty people are always such as eat too large a proportion of carbonaceous food, either butter, or the fat of meats, or fine flour, which is mostly starch, or sugar, or all combined—and sometimes all at a single meal. Of course they get too little phosphorus, not a particle of that element being found in fat, starch, or sugar, and are strongly predisposed to inflammations—always keeping the timber hot, especially if to these carbonaceous and heating articles of food are added the unnatural stimulus of alcoholic drinks.

Still, having wonderful powers of conforming to circumstances, Nature keeps the machine running comparatively well, till some excitement of mind or muscle exhausts the phosphorus below the point of endurance, and Nature cries out in agony for more vitality and less heat. The fuel being stopped the heat subsides, and after a few days, by heating up gradually, the machine will work again, till it is again overheated, and the exciting cause again renewed, to go through the same agony and the same process of temporary cure.

If the excitement which exhausts the phosphorus, and causes the fit of gout, be mental, the soda which is combined with phosphorus in the brain is set free, and, uniting with uric acid, forms the urate of soda, which constitutes the urinary calculi and the chalky deposits peculiar to gout. And it will probably be found that these deposits occur in gouty men of mental activity, and in fits of gout produced by mental excitement or mental exhaustion.

Again: gouty people are always sedentary in their habits; and here we get also a corroboration of the theory that want of phosphorus is the cause of gout. By reference to the tables of analyses of different articles of food, in Philosophy of Eating, pages 120–126, it will be seen that the phosphates and nitrates are always united, these articles containing the most muscle-making food, which contain the most phosphorus; and it will be seen also that those who exercise the muscles most require most nitrogenous food. Active men, therefore, require and will have more nitrogenous food than sedentary men, and with it get, of course, more phosphorus. And this explains the fact that laboring men never have the gout.

The only other peculiarity of gout usually mentioned is, that gentlemen, and not ladies, are most subject to it. But this, I think, is equally true of all inflammatory diseases, which are induced, not only by carbonaceous food, but by alcoholic drinks. And the explanation is this: gentlemen "tarry long at the wine" after the cloth is removed and the ladies are dismissed.

Dyspepsia, derangements of the stomach, bowels, &c., are all accounted for on the same principles, as is explained in the chapter on Dyspepsia, &c. My belief, therefore, is, that living according to the laws of life, as explained in Philosophy of Eating, no one, however predisposed to it, will ever have the gout. And if living otherwise he gets into its screws, the quickest way to get out of them is first to let off the steam, not by exhausting medicine, but by stopping the supply of fuel, and then restoring the nervous and vital equilibrium, by taking, in a form to be relished, food prepared from active fishes, birds, or animals, with bread or plain puddings from wheat, barley, or oatmeal, with cheese, as it can be well digested, and enough of butter, or other agreeable carbonates, to supply any deficiency of fat in the fish or lean meat, and to give relish to the food, and enough of some agreeable fruits or vegetables to furnish the necessary acids and waste which is wanting in cheese.

ADULTERATIONS OF FOOD, POISON FROM CULINARY UTENSILS, &c.

HAVING been frequently requested, by letter and verbally, to write a chapter on the diseases and symptoms produced by lead, copper, zinc, &c., as they are taken from water pipes, culinary vessels, fruit cans, &c., and used in cooking; and from phosphorus, soda, plaster of Paris, &c., which are used for raising bread, adulterating food, &c.; and to give some information as to the precautions necessary to avoid poisons in the various ways in which we are exposed to them, I will devote a few pages to that important subject.

And in order to ascertain the extent of the evils thus to be guarded against, I have requested Dr. S. Dana Hayes, our State Assayer, whose professional duties bring him in constant contact with them, to give me a list of cases of adulterations, poisoning from cooking utensils, &c., and he has kindly furnished me the following items: —

"*Flour* is hardly ever adulterated, but is frequently injured.

Meals the same.

Butter often contains lard and water in large proportions, and is colored.

Lard sometimes contains thirty-three per cent. of added water.

Sugar (especially brown) is often contaminated with iron, and thus colors tea or coffee brown or black.

Cream of Tartar and *Spices* are often adulterated with flour, meal, plaster, ground tan, &c.

Tea is seldom adulterated here, but sometimes old leaves, that have been used are re-dried and sold, mixed with good tea.

Coffee (ground) is very often impure and injured.

Milk the same.

Wines are very often made without any grapes.

Spirits often contain fusil oil and dissolved metals, such as copper and lead.

Vinegar often contains copper, lead, plaster, sulphuric acid, &c.

Soda Water frequently contains copper dissolved.

Chocolate, &c., generally pure and harmless.

Culinary Vessels often contaminate food with metallic poisons.

Lead and *Zinc* (galvanized) *Water Pipes* are frequently dissolved by drinking-water to such an extent as to become honey-combed. The presence of two different metals in water, tea, coffee, beer, &c., or the boiling or standing of such liquids in vessels made of two kinds of metal, and of joints in pipes, give rise to galvanic action, and the solution of one or both metals in the liquids to a dangerous extent. This galvanic action is far more common than is generally supposed, and a source of much ill health.

Arsenic often produces serious diseases, the air of sleeping-rooms being impregnated with it from the green of paper-hangings; and so sad and manifest are its effects from this cause, that in France it is a criminal offence, punishable by imprisonment, to use arsenic in coloring them.

Bread raised with saleratus and *cream of tartar* contains carbonic acid and tartrate of soda, or, if sour milk be used instead of cream of tartar, lactic of soda.

Bread raised with yeast contains carbonic acid gas; but on being exposed to the air, the gas is exchanged for pure air, and nothing injurious is left, unless the yeast be bad.

Aerated Bread contains nothing injurious.

Phosphatic Bread, or that which is raised by 'Horsford's Self-raising Bread Preparation,' which is composed of phosphoric acid and bi-carbonate of soda, contains, like other raised bread, carbonic acid gas, and also phosphate of soda, and some phosphate of lime."

The Effects on the System of different Poisons.

By accidental poisonings, and by scores and even hundreds of tests of the effects of all poisons in small quantities, each test being recorded by itself, homeopathic physicians can tell what symptoms to expect and what indeed are sure to come from taking any poison. But the effects are in very different degrees by different individuals; and as an assistance to housekeepers, to determine whether their families are receiving any poisonous effects from the sources suggested by Dr. Hayes, I will give the prominent symptoms produced on most people, but not on all, by long-continued influence from them in small doses, by each poison to which he refers.

Arsenic. The prominent effects of arsenic in small quantities, as reported, are: Sudden excessive debility, burning internal pains, convulsions, jaundice, general coldness, sleeplessness, painful stinging ulcers, blood blisters, startings and restlessness, excessive anxiety, vertigo, beating pain in the head, inflammation of the eyes, nausea and vomiting, cutting colic pains, itching and burning and painful eruptions on the skin, chilliness, followed by fever, sometimes periodical, great prostration.

Iron is the least poisonous of any of the metals; still it does produce manifest effects on the system, even in small quantities, taken for a long time. The most prominent are: General debility and emaciation, a sense of weariness and restlessness, loss of appetite, nose-bleed and other hemorrhages, pains in the chest, and cough; and, in the opinion of the celebrated Dr. Trousseau, it develops tubercles, and causes consumption, &c.

Copper. Pain in the bones, spasms or convulsions, epileptic fits, nausea and vomiting, painful sense of suffocation, ulcers and eruptions on the skin, paleness, pressure at the pit of the stomach, &c.

Lead. Weakness of the limbs, with dull, aching pain, and partial or general paralysis, bluish or yellowish paleness of the skin, drowsiness in the daytime, but sleeplessness at night, melancholy, excessive pain in the stomach and bowels, with obstinate costiveness, hoarseness, and sense of stricture of the throat, &c.

Tin. Emaciation, hysterical convulsions, paralysis, night sweats, burning heat in the limbs, inflamed eyelids, dimness of sight, heaviness and stupefying pressure on the head, sunken eyes, &c.

Lime, as it exists in plaster of Paris, is generally considered inert and harmless; but in that or any other form, lime, in small quantities, continuously taken, produces rheumatic pains in the limbs, swelling of the bones, nervous excitement, eruptions on the skin, headache, dizziness, yellow complexion, toothache, loss of appetite, constipation, dryness of the nose, palpitation, &c.

Soda and *Potash.* Constipation, pains in stomach and bowels, sour eructations, heartburn, wind, sense of distention, indigestion, &c.; in short, the symptoms which they are known to relieve, and for which they are so much taken. And hence it is always true of these, and all other crude medicines, in large doses, or small doses often repeated, that those who take them to relieve certain symptoms are sure to need them again soon; and thus every dose of any active medicine creates a demand for its repetition.

Zinc. Tearing pains in the limbs, painful soreness of the flesh, violent trembling of the whole body, heaviness and weariness, fretfulness and peevishness, dizziness, oppressive headache, pains in the face, like neuralgia and toothache, burning at the stomach, painful tension of the abdomen, pains in the back, vomiting, &c.

Carbonic Acid Gas. Burning pains in the stomach and bowels, with distention and flatulence, constipation, bitter taste in the mouth, water-brash, heartburn, restlessness and sleeplessness at night, chilliness, itching of the skin, nettlerash, boils and ulcers, pain in the head, with nausea or sick headache, sense of weakness in the limbs, and the limbs go to sleep. Some or all of these symptoms are experienced generally by those who eat newly-made bread raised with yeast or yeast powders, as the cells of the bread are filled with this gas; but after standing in the air for a few hours the gas is exchanged for pure air. And the same troubles are experienced by those who drink effervescing beers, or wines, or soda water, or anything else that contains this gas.

Phosphorus and *Phosphoric Acid.* Soreness and swelling of the bones and joints, *caries, or decay of the bones*, emaciation, boils and itching ulcers, fine rash pimples, yellow teeth, hoarseness, tickling cough, cough with purulent expectorations, loss of voice, *impotence*, *consumption*, &c. All these symptoms, except those printed in Italics, and many more distressing, have been repeatedly produced by taking phosphorus, or the acid, which produces the same effect, in quantities much smaller than those taken daily in bread from "Horsford's Self-raising Bread Preparation;" and those in Italics, terminating in death or the destruction of the bones, have been produced by working in an atmosphere impregnated with them in a match factory. The other ingredient in the Horsford's Self-raising Bread Preparation, according to the label on each package, is pure bi-carbonate of soda, which, according to an established law, does not neutralize the evil effects of the phosphorus, but adds to them its own deleterious effects, some of which are as follows: —

Bi-carbonate of Soda. Indigestion, chronic debility, pressure at the stomach after eating, flatulence, distention of stomach and bowels, headache, blotches on the skin, toothache, vertigo, twitching in sleep, &c., which, being added to the symptoms produced by phosphoric acid, will make an imperfect list of the evils which may be expected from the common use of this preparation.

Another fact that enhances the danger of this "bread preparation," is, that its principal elements are mineral, and, like all other mineral elements, its poisonous effects are insidious and cumulative; and, as men will sometimes drink of water impregnated with lead for years without suspecting danger, and then become hopelessly diseased by its influence, so they may take this more deadly poison without suspecting danger till it is too late to escape death from it.

I knew a young man who worked for years in a match factory, without suspecting danger, when all at once a fatal disease of the lungs supervened to all the symptoms of phosphorus, which soon carried him off.

And, what may be considered a worse calamity, the bones — especially, for reasons not yet understood, those of the face — become diseased, and decay, producing the most loathsome condition that can be imagined. Such cases frequently occur where no danger was suspected till too late.

The danger is also enhanced by the position of the inventor and manufacturer. I have known a number of instances in which people have left comparatively innocent modes of bread making, and have taken up this, because it is recommended by a Professor of Harvard College; and finding out their dangerous mistake, some have written to the Professor, and explaining the arguments against it, asking his explanation.

His answer to one intelligent gentleman was sent to me; but it is mislaid, and I quote it from memory: "I have not time to go fully into the explanation; but it is sufficient to say that Liebig, the greatest living chemist, has taught nothing incompatible with my theory." The gentleman was not satisfied with the explanation, and returned, as every sensible man would, to his unleavened bread, and to that made with fresh yeast.

I have read, I believe, all the principal works of Liebig, and it does not appear that he ever gave a thought to the principle, which clearly explains the ground of the Professor's terrible mistake, viz., that of which Dr. Hayes says, in the quotation before referred to, "Modern investigations *certainly* sustain the ground taken (in the Philosophy of Eating) that organized elements are the only ones assimilated in the human system."

If Liebig had gone into these investigations he would have seen at once that phosphorus obtained from calcined bones must be poisonous, according to the law of Nature, which supplies this important element only organized in grains and the flesh of animals, and makes all other forms of it poisonous. The ground which Dr. Hayes says is *certainly sustained*, is this: "Before the mountains were brought forth," God instituted laws by which all the phosphorus, and iron, and all other elements which were to constitute the human system, or should ever be needed to keep it in repair, should be organized in the vegetable kingdom, and should be stored there, and in the flesh of animals which live on vegetables; so that wherever man chooses to live, he finds all these elements prepared for him.

And to prevent us from resorting to any other source of supply, he at the same time instituted a law, making it impossible that a particle of them should be assimilated or used in the system, and making all elements not thus organized poisons, more or less virulent according to their importance in the system. Under this law phosphorus made from calcined bones cannot, of course, be assimilated; but being one of the most important elements in the system, is made the most virulent poison.

Here the learned Professor joins issue with his Maker, and under a patent from the government of the United States, directly infringing on the patent issued by the Government of Heaven and Earth, with penalties for infringement truly appalling, as we have seen, he sows the seeds of death among the people, with the following extraordinary, not to say false, statement of facts, printed on every package of his phosphatic bread-raising powders: —

After recounting the evils produced by soda, cream of tartar, and other bread-raising materials, which are mere trifles compared with those produced by phosphorus, he says, "How then shall we make good bread? Professor Horsford has given to the world a scientific solution of this great problem in domestic economy; and the Self-raising Bread Preparation, manufactured under his patent and direction, has met the *unqualified approval of every physician* and *chemist* and *physiologist* who has examined and tried it"! "It is a *simple phosphate*, and *nearly restores* to the flour the *essential* and *nutritive properties* removed with the bran — *nothing else*"!

These statements, made as they are in the very teeth of Divine testimony, and contradicting, as they do, the direct testimony of scientific men standing at least as high as himself, — two of whom have told him, to my knowledge, that they considered his phosphatic bread preparation a poison, — certainly must deceive many innocent people, and lead them into destruction of health and life. This fatal mistake comes from ignoring the vital law, to which chemical law is always subservient as lower law to higher. The principle is clearly recognized by Dr. Hayes, as already quoted.

"Modern investigation certainly sustains the ground taken (in the "Philosophy of Eating"), that organized elements only are assimilated in the human system." Phosphorus, therefore, to be assimilated, must be taken as organized in natural food. If disorganized, as in Professor Horsford's phosphatic yeast powders, it is poison. This, I assert, not only on the authority of nature's clearly revealed law, but on the authority of every physiological chemist, so far as I know, who recognizes vital law as superior to chemical law. On this point I can furnish the names of our most eminent physiological chemists. Dr. J. Francis Churchill quotes from Dr. Buckheim, a celebrated chemist who has given particular attention to vital chemistry, as endorsing the opinion of four other celebrated German chemists in regard to the very form of phosphoric acid and soda used in the phosphatic powders in question as follows: "Woehler and Frenich, basing their opinion as much upon their own experiments as upon those of Weigel and Krug, have concluded that phosphoric acid has a poisonous effect analogous to arsenic." "The same also holds good with the phosphatic salts of soda." *

* Those analytical chemists who sustain Professor Horsford in the assertion that his preparation "nearly restores to the flour the essential and nutritive properties removed with the bran," entirely ignore this vital law, and take for granted that which every physiologist knows to be untrue, that chemical agents act in the stomach as they act in retorts. To sustain my position I have the promise of the names of some of our most distinguished chemists and physiologists in this country, but the press cannot wait, and I must use them, if necessary, in some other way.

GALVANIC ACTION PRODUCES POISON FROM CULINARY VESSELS.

THAT is certainly an important fact referred to by Dr. Hayes, that galvanic action produces poison from water pipes and culinary vessels; and its principles ought to be explained, that its evils may be avoided. (See Philosophy of Eating, page 200.) Let us try to explain the conditions necessary to produce this effect.

What produces galvanic action? If any one will take two small pieces of different metals, say a copper cent and a silver quarter, or copper and zinc, perfectly clean and tasteless, and place one over and the other under the tongue, so that no part of the one shall touch the other, he will perceive no taste or sensible effect; but if he bring the edges of each piece together, so as to touch at any point, immediately will he perceive a strong taste of one or both of the metals, and perhaps a slight twinge of pain. This is galvanic action, or a particular development of electricity, and this shows the conditions necessary to produce it. Two metals connected at least at one point, but no matter how intimately, must both be moistened by some liquid, and if the liquid be salt or acid the effect will be stronger.

Many of our culinary utensils have two metals connected, as pans with tin tops and copper bottoms, or tin soldered with lead, which tin is itself iron with a tin coating; or stew-pans of iron coated with zinc or tin, &c., as are also water pipes, coated with zinc or tin, or soldered at their joints, or attached to a copper pump. These are more or less active batteries according to the amount of metal thus united, the extent to which it is exposed to the liquid, and the character of the liquid—whether acid, or salt, or pure.

Copper and also galvanized iron pumps are powerful batteries, affecting the taste of the water in them in a very few minutes, especially if the water be hard. So is also a large boiler, partly tin and partly copper, or any vessel with the bottom of one metal and the top of another. But the most dangerous battery to which families in the country are exposed is *zinc or tin-coated lead pipe*, which, when the coating is imperfect, as it generally is, is honey-combed in a few months, especially if the water be hard, the lead and zinc both being dissolved in the water. Tin cans for fruits, unless the tin is good, and the coating so perfect that the iron is not exposed to the acid juice ât any one point, and unless made tight without solder, must have some influence on the juice of the fruit. Soda fountains, being made of different metals, and their contents being active salts, are quite effective batteries, and undoubtedly impregnate the soda with their metallic poisons.

But the most powerful galvanic battery, and that to the deleterious influence of which city people are most exposed, is formed of a large copper boiler in the kitchen, connected by three or four coils of lead pipe to a large zinc-lined cistern in the attic.

Here is a battery, affecting all the water in the cistern, boiler, and the lead pipes intervening, impregnating it every moment with dissolved lead, copper, and zinc, and causing in those who use the water the combined pains and cumulative diseases which these three most poisonous metals are known to produce.

It is true that Cochituate, Croton, Schuylkill, and Mystic waters, with which Boston, New York, Philadelphia, and Charlestown are supplied, and the waters with which cities generally are supplied, are so nearly pure as to have much less galvanic influence than hard waters.

But remembering the fact referred to, that a clean cent and a clean silver quarter, with less than an inch of surface each, moistened by the pure juices of the tongue of the purest mouth, will produce a sufficient effect to give a distinct and instantaneous taste of copper and silver; and remembering that a galvanic battery has power to dissolve metals in proportion to the extent of the surface of the metals composing it, and that we get the influence of this vast extent of surface of copper of the boiler, lead sometimes of all the pipes in the house, and zinc on the whole surface of the cistern, and we cannot fail to realize that the influence must be appalling, even with soft water. Indeed, we know that copper boilers are constantly requiring repairs, the lead pipe, especially about the soldered joints, constantly rusting into holes and leaking, and the cistern always coated with a white crust of salts of zinc.

The danger from this influence is much less in some houses than others. Some have no cistern, and therefore have a less powerful battery and none of the deleterious influence of zinc. Some have service pipes connected directly with the pipes of the street, and can get water that is not subject to this galvanic influence by keeping it carefully drawn out of the service pipes before use for the family.

Others get all the water through the cistern, the pipes all going into it, and the water all going into the galvanic circle before it can be drawn; but on inquiring, as I always do, for water to use with medicine, directly from the street, I find not one housekeeper in ten who can tell whether the water in any particular part of the house comes from the cistern or not. They are generally, but not always, afraid of warm water that comes from the copper boiler, and that is the extent of their care on that subject.

If the water used in cooking or drinking comes directly from the street pipes, there is no great danger, with care always to draw off, before using it, all the water that stands in the service pipes; but water within the galvanic circle, such as has been explained, cannot be drawn pure. This may be inferred from the fact that, in the experiment with the cent and the silver quarter, the taste of the copper and silver is instantaneously produced when the edges of the metals touch each other, and continues as long as they remain in contact.

Ice-Pitchers. Another source of poison from galvanic action, of no inconsiderable consequence, is water standing in ice-pitchers. Until lately, to protect them from injury by ice falling into them, the bottoms were made of a thick layer of a cheaper metal, which forms, with the top, a battery that is constantly dissolving one or all the different metals of which it is composed, and the action is so great as to cause them to be constantly leaking, till the trouble of keeping them in repair, rather than the danger of poison, has brought into use pitchers made only of one metal, or, what is better, unless made without solder, a metal surrounding a glass pitcher, which is absolutely safe.

Cooking utensils, made of one metal, either of iron, copper, zinc, or block tin, if kept clean, impart no deleterious influence to food in the common modes of cooking; but in making pickles, with vinegar, in copper kettles, to give them a good green color; in making lemonade in tubs and buckets painted with white lead; in keeping acid sauces, preserved acid fruits, pickles, &c., in earthen jars glazed with a preparation of lead; besides the various other sources of poison to which I have referred, families are constantly exposed to the influence of some dissolved metal. And when we consider how much suffering one dissolved metal causes, the wonder is not that, with systems debilitated as they are with the use of unnatural food, we suffer so much sickness and lose so many of our children, but rather that we enjoy any degree of health, or live long enough to perpetuate the race.

THE GRECIAN BEND.

BEING accidentally in a popular store on Washington Street, and seeing the clerks rush to the window, with the exclamation, "O, my!" my attention was called to an elegantly-dressed young lady in the street, doing the exquisite on the Grecian bend. She was evidently a disciple of the English dressmaker and authoress referred to (page 103), who, in order to restore the old spider-waist fashion, recommends that the waists of genteel young ladies should never be allowed to measure but fifteen inches in circumference — that is, five inches in diameter.

I had never before seen a genuine Grecian bend, excepting in the monkey begging for pennies for his master, and the little dog asking for a bit of bread; and the resemblance in the cases seemed to me remarkable, not only on account of the motives which induced the ridiculous attitude (in which, by the way, the dog and the monkey had the advantage, they aiming at substantial good, while she sought only admiration), but in the peculiar waddle of gait with which they progressed. And I said to myself, "What can be the philosophy of this remarkable resemblance?" On reflection, I think the explanation is anatomical. Ladies, being intended to walk erect, have hip-joints so constructed that they move smoothly and gracefully only in that position, while those joints in quadrupeds are constructed to move smoothly while in the horizontal position. In assuming the Grecian bend, therefore, the joints of both quadrupeds and bipeds are out of place alike, and the waddling motion is, of course, alike in each.

She waddled a few rods past the store, and then turned round, smiling, or rather smirking, complacently on her "crowd of admirers," with an expression of face which seemed to say, with the correspondent of the author referred to, "All my torture is repaid by the admiration I excite." And I wanted to quote the apostrophe of Burns to the louse:—

"O, wad some power the giftie gie us
To see oursels as ithers see us!
It wad frae monie a blunder free us
An' foolish notion:
What airs in dress an' gait wad lea'e us,
And e'en devotion!"

The silly thing had probably read the book referred to, in which is said to be repeated, three or four times, the slander on all men of common sense, "Men admire taper waists," and had conceived the ridiculous idea that men also admire the monkey waddle; but I wish that she, and all other addle-headed girls who are bent on deformity (pardon the miserable pun), could know what those sensible young men did think of her, and what all sensible men, young or old, think of such, or any attempts to improve the natural gait or form.

One of them asked me to write a chapter on the Grecian Bend; but the chapter in which it belongs being already printed, I can only follow the example of the renowned Lord Timothy Dexter, who placed his commas, semi-colons, colons, &c., on a page of his book by themselves, with the request that each reader should "pepper according to his own taste." This article being intended for condiment only, may be used in like manner to spice any dull article, according to the discretion of the reader; but it properly belongs with the consideration of other deformations (page 101).

THE PHILOSOPHY OF EATING.

THE public appreciation of this book, to which the "HOW NOT TO BE SICK" is a sequel, is seen by the fact that, with very little advertising, the fourth edition is demanded within the first nine months of its publication. Its object and character are well defined by the PACIFIC MEDICAL AND SURGICAL JOURNAL, one of the best medical journals in the country: "The character of it is denoted by its title. It belongs to the same class of compositions as that excellent production, Johnston's Chemistry of Common Life. It is not a medical work, though it embodies a vast amount of knowledge not ordinarily found outside the limits of medical literature. Without any qualifications or misgivings, we commend it, with great satisfaction, to the general reader."

By an analysis of the composition of the human system, and showing what elements are used every day in muscular and mental labor, and what are used in furnishing animal heat; and by analyses of the different kinds of food in common use, we ascertain where to get the necessary elements in natural food, and what we lose in butter, fine flour, &c.

How we lose the best elements of wheat, and how Nature provides for more heating food in cold climates than warm, are seen in the cuts below, which were taken from this book:—

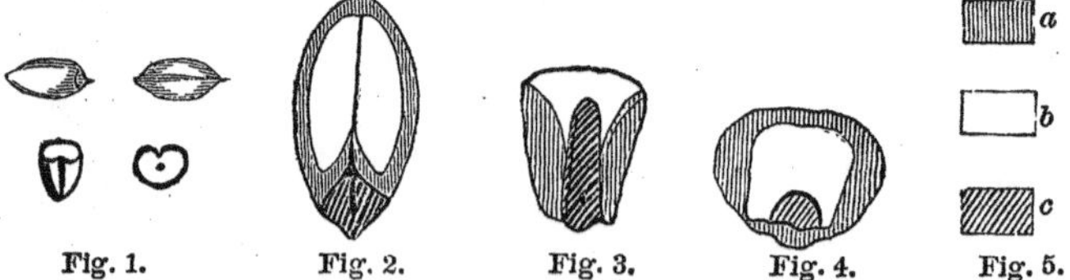

Fig. 1. Fig. 2. Fig. 3. Fig. 4. Fig. 5.

Fig. 1.—Wheat of natural size.
Fig. 2.—Wheat magnified.
Fig. 3.—Southern corn. } Showing the different proportions of nutritive
Fig. 4.—Northern corn. } elements in each, as explained page 25.

a The muscle-making elements.
b The heat or fat producers.
c The food for brains and nerves.

We have received from literary men, editors, &c., over two hundred voluntary testimonials, of which the following are samples: —

HARRIET BEECHER STOWE: "It is a very much needed work, and it strikes me as written in a very clear, popular style, and conveying much truth for which *human nature is perishing*." "There is an absolute *demand* for a book on the plan of yours, and yours strikes me as placing these much needed ideas in a very clear light." "As to the controverted points, I am, of course, no judge. I can only say, Well said, perfectly clear and intelligible, and important, if true."

DR. S. DANA HAYES, State Assayer of Massachusetts, says of the principal controverted points referred to by Mrs. Stowe: "Modern investigations *certainly* sustain the ground taken, that organized elements are the only ones assimilated in the human system."

EPES SARGENT, ESQ., says to the same point: "The facts are, I believe, in accordance with the discoveries of the most advanced chemical and anatomical science, and are very suggestive." "Certainly the long attention of the author to chemistry, in its relations to food, must have qualified him to speak with authority on these points."

JOEL MARBLE, ESQ., who for thirty years was principal of academies and provider for boarding-scholars, says: "It presents a common-sense system, that can be put into practice by every family. Such a help to me would have been invaluable. If he who makes two blades of grass grow where but one grew before is a benefactor to his race, what shall he be called who adds months and years to men's lives, and makes those lives healthier and happier?"

DR. FROST, of Philadelphia, writes: "It is filled with valuable and most important information."

The LONDON BOOKSELLER says: "It takes much higher ground than any popular volume of the kind in England." "It discusses, and that in the most entertaining fashion, the wants and resources of the human body, the elements of animal and vegetable food, and their adaptation to the requirements of the animal man."

GILBERT HAVEN, D. D., Editor of Zion's Herald, says: "It examines, in a thorough, scholarly, and practical manner, the composition of our daily food, shows what errors prevail in our national diet, and how they can be corrected." "Every family should possess a copy."

The BOSTON JOURNAL says: "One of the most practically useful books that has been issued from the press for a long time." "For the scientific accuracy of his theories he has good authority — for most of them he has, at least, the support of common sense."

The DOVER STAR says: "The amount of information crowded between these covers is immense."

WILLIAM HAGUE, D. D., says: "There are thousands, no doubt, in every walk of life, who would acknowledge their indebtedness to the author for expositions so lucid, so minute, and so well harmonizing the plainest practical rules with the latest advancements of science."

The BURLINGTON FREE PRESS says: "It is not one of the '*death in the pot*' treatises which forbid everything palatable in the shape of food, but is a scientific and sensible work."

The CINCINNATI ADVOCATE says: "It will be health in your stomach, muscle in your body, clearness in your brain, as well as money in your purse, to send to the nearest bookseller, and read and heed its wholesome suggestions."

The NEW ENGLAND FARMER says: "There would be little need of a physician, or of medicines, were this book widely circulated."

The FREE PRESS says: "We welcome the volume as one that will furnish really substantial, practical, and reliable information; and if properly studied, and its precepts followed, will be of untold value."

The NATION says: "A much needed work, written in a very clear and pleasant style, embracing three very important questions, — What shall we eat? How shall we eat? and When shall we eat? It should find a place in every household."

The HARTFORD COURANT says: "This book ought to have a wide circulation, for it cannot fail to do good." "It is throughout intelligent, and is admirably arranged."

The DETROIT POST says: "The subject is treated in familiar language, and so illustrated and enforced by plain, sound advice as to health and living, that it forms an excellent companion, not to say substitute, for the family medicine-books."

www.ingramcontent.com/pod-product-compliance
Lightning Source LLC
LaVergne TN
LVHW021251110826
845151LV00002BA/383

* 9 7 8 1 4 2 5 5 3 9 1 9 1 *